WHEN DREAMS COME TRUE

ABOUT THE AUTHOR

Rosanna Davison is author of *Eat Yourself Fit* and the No. 1 bestseller *Eat Yourself Beautiful*. She is a qualified nutritional therapist with a Master of Science degree in Personalised Nutrition. She leapt to global prominence at the age of 19 when she was crowned Miss World 2003 in China. In the years since earning that accolade, she has enjoyed a busy international career as a model, writer and media personality.

WHEN DREAMS COME TRUE

THE HEARTBREAK AND HOPE ON
MY JOURNEY TO MOTHERHOOD

ROSANNA DAVISON

GILL BOOKS

Gill Books
Hume Avenue
Park West
Dublin 12
www.gillbooks.ie

Gill Books is an imprint of M.H. Gill and Co.

978 07171 91833

Designed by Bartek Janczak
Edited by Alison Walsh
Copyedited by Emma Dunne
Proofread by Sally Vince

Printed by ScandBook AB, Sweden
This book is typeset in 11.5 on 17.5pt, Sabon.

A CIP catalogue record for this book is available from the
British Library.

5 4 3 2 1

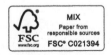

To my wonderful husband, Wesley, and my parents, Diane and Chris, thank you for your unwavering love, support and encouragement.

To my children, Sophia, Hugo and Oscar, this book is for you. I love you beyond words, for ever and always.

CONTENTS

INTRODUCTION

My aim in writing this book about our struggles with fertility – the long and challenging surrogacy journey we undertook to have our daughter, Sophia, followed by the joy of welcoming naturally conceived identical twin boys less than a year later – is to help normalise the conversation about infertility and pregnancy loss. I feel that sharing my story about the frustration and loneliness I experienced as we struggled to have a family may encourage others to speak out about their difficulties. Contributing to the growing conversation about miscarriage will hopefully help us to realise that it's an experience sadly shared by many people and hiding it only further stigmatises pregnancy loss and infertility. By sharing the heartbreak and hope on my path to motherhood, I hope to give others struggling with fertility issues or even new parenthood the comfort and support to feel less alone on what can be a difficult and traumatic road.

I understand that for so many of you on your own fertility journeys your family dream hasn't yet come true. You may still be in the midst of it, feeling emotionally and physically drained. Perhaps you're starting to believe that it'll never happen, that your chance to hold your much-wanted baby is dwindling with each month and year that passes. Or maybe you're struggling with intense guilt and self-blame for not being able to have a baby. I know exactly how that feels because I experienced disappointment and loss month after month and began to despair of my 'broken' body as I struggled through fourteen early miscarriages and a shock fifteenth pregnancy loss at just over ten weeks, before discovering that I was expecting our boys, Hugo and Oscar, only six weeks later.

Today, I'm a proud mother of three beautiful children aged one and under. They were born just under a year apart and together they've changed our lives in the best possible way. I wrote this book for Sophia, Hugo and Oscar to read in the future so they'll know how they came into the world, how much we longed for them and how deeply loved they are. I hope that they'll show it to their children, and perhaps their grandchildren will one day read our story of love, loss, hope and a family dream come true.

CHAPTER 1

SLIDING DOORS

I feel extremely lucky to be able to say that I had a very happy, normal childhood with my two younger brothers, Michael and Hubert, or Hubie as we know him. My dad spent months away on the road and we'd go with him sometimes when he was touring Europe – we even joined him on tours in Australia and Canada – but my mum, Diane, made sure that we were sheltered from certain aspects of the music business. We weren't spoiled and had as regular a life as possible. We have a strong work ethic that comes from both of our parents, who have always worked hard. They encouraged us to study and to work for our independence. We still had to do our chores on a Saturday morning and behave well! We were an outdoor-loving, sporty family and also spent a lot of our younger childhoods running around the garden playing with Milly, our much-loved black Labrador, and I really want my own children to have the same kind of carefree experience packed with adventures. The focus was on family, spending as much time as possible outdoors and, apart from watching Saturday-morning cartoons while snuggled up under a duvet on the sitting-room sofa, we had very little screen time. We had wonderful holidays in my grandparents' home, Bargy Castle in Wexford, where we helped on the farm and had great fun paddling and later swimming in the sea at the local beaches. Some of my happiest childhood memories are from my time spent on the farm with my grandmother. I'm incredibly grateful that my children have a great-grandmother and I hope to keep her memory alive for them in the future through this book and my own recollections.

I was always most content in my wellies and old waxed jacket, helping her during lambing season. The lambing pens were affectionately referred to as 'Shepherd's Hotel' and there was usually a pen in the yard for orphaned or poorly lambs who needed extra care and attention. I used to love helping my granny prepare bottles for feeding the lambs by hand. In fact, prepping Sophia's bottles by mixing cooled boiled water with scoops of powdered formula brought all of those memories flooding back.

As a horse-mad child and teenager, I pestered my mum

to buy me the pony magazines in our local newsagent's and dreamed of one day owning my own pony. I loved my weekly horse-riding lessons, competed in hunter trials and showjumping events on friends' ponies, enjoyed long blissful summers at pony camp and read every equine book I could get my hands on. Granny even bred racehorses at one point during her incredibly interesting life, before building up a herd of Aberdeen Angus cattle with an Aberdeen bull she persuaded her farmhand Billy to lead around the parade ring in order to win competitions. She ran Bargy Castle as a hotel with my grandfather Charles Davison from the early 1960s until the late '80s, doing all the cooking for guests, buying produce and running the farm. I only discovered in my mid-twenties, through filming an episode of *Who Do You Think You Are?* for RTÉ, that they had spent some time together in Malta in the 1950s working in espionage during the Cold War. Like a storyline straight out of a James Bond thriller, their Maltese mission was to train young Albanians to work as spies and experts in destruction by means of explosives, to enable them to overturn the tyrannical communist government in Albania.

I'm in awe of my granny's strength and stoicism, and I love to hear her colourful stories from her time spent playing polo in Lagos in the 1950s or her early life in India, but we've bonded most over our shared love of horses. As a family, we spent much of our summer holidays, and Easter and Halloween mid-term breaks, down in Wexford at Littlebridge, my parents' farmhouse adjacent to Bargy Castle. I have many wonderful memories of long hazy days running among the golden hay bales, Easter-egg hunts under frothy cherry blossoms and autumnal bonfire nights toasting marshmallows, our breath visible in the frosty air.

One rainy night in early November 1996, we had just finished supper in the warm and spacious old-fashioned kitchen at Bargy when Granny suggested we take a walk down the yard to the stables, where she promised that a surprise was waiting. At just twelve years old, I was perplexed. But, after wrapping up against the cold, I grabbed a torch and we walked down towards the farm outbuildings. As a floodlight lit up the yard, I heard the unmistakable shrill whinny of a pony ringing out across the cobbles. 'But what is a horse doing here?' I thought while I walked closer to investigate. I peered into the murky darkness of the stable and saw a dark, shiny eyeball staring back at me as the bay mare moved closer towards the half-door. 'She's for you to try out if you'd like to?' Granny smiled at me. My very own pony! It was the moment I had been dreaming of since my aunt Sarah had brought me for my first horse-riding lesson at the age of seven.

Granny had arranged with a friend to buy the Welsh mare, whom I named Molly, and for her to be cared for at Bargy when I couldn't be there to groom and exercise her. But I spent most weekends with Molly at Bargy, enjoying long hacks across the fields, exploring little lanes and forests, setting up jumps with a long plank of wood across two oil drums and entering as many local gymkhanas as I could. Later on, I would take the train from Dublin to Wexford and stay with Granny in the castle. I used to spend hours carefully polishing Molly's saddle and bridle, plaiting her mane and tail, grooming her glistening coat and painting hoof oil onto her hooves, before Granny would help me to load her into the horse-box and drive me to various competitions in the area. In hindsight, I probably caused her and my parents plenty of worry with my fearless exploits. During the summer of '97, I entered us into a local hunter trials competition, designed to test the ability of horse and rider to jump a series of natural fences and obstacles. I loved the speed and thrill of a cross-country course, and all was going well until we reached the coffin jump. Molly stumbled as she attempted to clear the fence and I was thrown off, landing heavily on my left shoulder, hand awkwardly bent back. Later that day, my whole hand swelled up, but it was only after I played a tennis match the following morning that it began to feel really painful. Mum drove me to Wexford Hospital and an X-ray diagnosed a hairline fracture. I was devastated to be told to avoid horse-riding for three weeks, but the day the cast came off I was back in the saddle.

I enjoyed four blissful years with Molly and many wonderful adventures, from summer pony camps to bareback sunset beach hacks and dips in the ocean. She was just thirteen hands tall so I sadly grew too big for her, and when I was sixteen Granny found a horse called Walnut. We decided to keep Molly as a companion for Walnut and, later, Granny sourced a suitable sire to put her into foal. She gave birth the following year to a gorgeous dun colt foal we named Harley Davison, and he was later sold to a Swedish family. Walnut and I enjoyed many fun moments too, and she was a wonderful jumper – most of the time. I remember on one occasion attempting a huge fence with Walnut at a show-jumping event. As she lifted her front hooves, she clipped the pole and lost her balance, causing her to lunge sideways and crash into the left-hand standard. I toppled off her and she rolled right over me. We both stood up, dazed and shocked but unhurt, as a crowd of people came rushing over to check on us. The experience didn't stop me from horse-riding but it gave Granny a fright, as she witnessed the accident from where she had been standing on the sidelines, cheering and clapping me on.

Granny has always been hugely encouraging and support-ive towards me and my brothers, so we love to make her feel special and appreciated. She celebrated her ninety-fourth birthday on 22 June 2020, and Hubie, Michael and I each wrote a letter for her with a selection of our favourite mem-ories of happy times spent with her.

Dear Granny,
As we celebrate your ninety-fourth birthday, I'm delighted to share some special memories of you from my childhood,

teenage and adult life to illustrate just how important you are to us as a family, the enormous impact you have had and continue to have on our lives and how much you've helped to shape and encourage our hobbies and interests.

As a little girl with a big love for animals, helping you around the farm was a huge highlight of my year, and I have so many fond memories of lambing season. I was by your side as you attended to sick ewes or orphaned lambs and your animals clearly adored you, as anytime I wore your battered old waxed jacket, they would gather around with huge excitement, pawing and nibbling at it, thinking that I was you! I almost have too many wonderful memories of horse-riding at Bargy through my teenage years to describe, but I'll never forget the tears of joy and magical excitement of having my very own pony and the many times you drove us to pony camps and gymkhanas around Wexford using your horse-box. It was such a special time for us, enjoying our mutual passion for horses.

Many of my other distinctive childhood memories of spending time with you at Bargy involve food – especially your delicious scones and coffee cakes, and the smell of sizzling sausages in the kitchen as you cooked breakfast for Hubie and Michael. And not to forget, more recently, your appreciation for the chips and the porridge on our family holidays in Mauritius. Having you on holiday with us for those years was really special for all of us, and it was wonderful to see how much you enjoyed the warmth, relaxation *and swimming in the sea. Sharing the excitement with you of getting engaged in January 2013 and the subsequent 'Champagne Sunday' celebrations is a great memory to have. You always loved making birthdays really memorable for us and went to great efforts to decorate the special birthday throne with pretty flowers. So many happy birthdays were celebrated in the kitchen at Bargy.*

Wes and I always love our visits to Littlebridge and Bargy for weekends, and the time we spend sitting chatting with you, either out at lunch, by the fireside over a cup of tea in the sitting room or with a gin and tonic outside on the sunny patio. I know Wes adores being offered a sweet treat from your choccy stash. A favourite visit was on 20 July 2019, when we told you that you had a new great-granddaughter on the way, and then you met Sophia for the first time on 27 December. We've shared many laughs and funny stories and look forward to plenty more visits once it's safe to see you again. We definitely need to stock you up again with hot chocolates!

Thank you for being such an important and special part of all of our lives. Wishing you a birthday filled with love, laughter and yummy cake, and many more happy returns.

Lots of love always,

Rosanna x

Above all, I'm deeply grateful for the kind of carefree, innocent childhood that my brothers and I had, and for all of the love and support we received from the people in our lives. I grew up with constant encouragement from my parents, which gave me the strength and self-confidence that I could do anything I wanted to once I worked hard at it and believed in myself and my abilities. One day, during a chat about my children, my dad shared his own approach to parenting: 'Surround them with so much love that it makes them strong enough for whatever life brings.' I feel that has really stood to me in the various experiences and challenges that I've faced in life and it's what I hope to do for Sophia, Hugo and Oscar too.

During summer 2003, in the old Dún Laoghaire shopping centre of all places, my life as I knew it changed. It was serendipity, a casual meeting, but I suppose that's how many of the important things in life happen, almost without you noticing them. Sometimes I wonder what might have transpired had I not made a particular choice and said yes to one thing and no to another, but that's life, isn't it? I have no regrets whatsoever and feel that I've been so lucky. At the time I was a first-year student in UCD, studying history of art and sociology. I was always more interested in human physiology, nutrition and sports science, but I couldn't find a course in Dublin that really appealed, so I was persuaded to opt for a more general degree first. I'm glad I did it, although if I were to have the opportunity again, I'd spend more time thinking about what I would like to achieve. At the age of eighteen, you think you have all the time in the world and that you can always do something else, but as I've realised with a shock, the years really begin to speed past!

So, there I was, aged nineteen, queueing at the ATM to withdraw money for a €10 top I'd spotted, when I heard a voice behind me say, 'Excuse me?'

I turned around to see a woman I didn't recognise. I thought she was looking for directions or the time until she said, 'I'm scouting for girls to enter Miss Dún Laoghaire and the competition is this Saturday night. Would you have any interest in entering?'

I'd never even heard of Miss Dún Laoghaire, and beauty pageants definitely didn't appeal, so I replied, 'No, sorry, I don't think it's for me.'

She said, 'Oh, please, we're short of entrants and there'll be free food and drink! And you can bring your friends. It'll be a good night out.' She was persuasive and eventually I agreed, having no idea what I was letting myself in for.

I turned up a few nights later in just a nice top, jeans and heels – the staple going-out outfit back then. I'm generally comfortable with meeting new people and make friends easily, but I remember arriving at the venue with butter-flies in my stomach and a sense of nervous anticipation at embarking on the unknown. I had taken part in the UCD fashion show in March of that year and had learned a lot about being on stage and projecting an air of confidence, and I had been taught how to stand up straight, keep my shoulders down and walk properly thanks to the wonderful coaching and choreography by Julian Benson. But I wasn't used to having all eyes on me, and the thought of that scared me a little. I generally took a very simple approach with my hair and make-up, so hadn't done much with either, apart from blow-drying my hair and applying a bit of mascara and lip gloss. Thankfully, it wasn't too intimidating, just a little competition in a nightclub bar; I had to walk the catwalk and answer a few questions from the judges, as well as have my photo taken.

To my utter shock, I won it. I couldn't believe it. My mother is my biggest supporter and she'd wanted to come and cheer me on with my little brother Michael and a friend, but at the time the boys were under-age, so they weren't allowed in. When she came and collected me later, I proudly showed her my tiara and sash with 'Miss Dún Laoghaire' printed on it in bold blue letters. I'd had a bit of fun, met some nice people and that was that, or so I thought.

I was very focused on my studies so I didn't want anything to stop me from finishing my degree and following it up with a master's. What I hadn't realised was that I would be put forward automatically for the Miss Ireland competition that summer. As it was planned to be held in August, I wouldn't miss any college and, that time, I took it a bit more seriously. I picked out a long sequinned dress and even had my first spray tan. The competition took place on a Friday night, which was at the end of my third week working in a school summer camp teaching art. At the beginning of that week I'd told my mum that I planned to take the Friday off work and have my hair and nails done. She told me I couldn't just take time off when I'd agreed to work and that, anyhow, I could easily do my own hair and nails. I still took the day off!

As far as I knew, there were no such things as hair extensions, fake nails or lash extensions in those days, and I wasn't particularly interested in beauty. I'd never really thought about being attractive or otherwise. I've always been much more interested in sports and fitness, so my general look was pretty casual. There's much more focus now on image, and social media has played a huge part in that. I didn't join social media until after I finished college, and I feel really grateful that I grew up in an era without camera phones and the often intense pressure and judgement that social media can bring. Back then, there was hardly even email – I would get faxes with details of jobs. And even though I appreciated fashion and dressing up in nice clothes for work, getting highlights was about as far as I went.

So when I won Miss Ireland in August 2003, it came as quite a shock. There had been a big build-up to the competition, with various TV and media commitments, photo calls and interviews. It was an incredibly exciting experience, although one that I had presumed would be short-lived. I had really enjoyed the whole process and made friends with some of the other contestants, but I genuinely didn't believe I had a hope of winning the competition, which was held in the ballroom at Dublin's City West Hotel. On the morning of the event, I vividly remember checking into my hotel room to begin preparing for the daytime interviews and feeling utterly petrified. What on earth was I doing there? I thought. My whole body shook throughout the interviews as I was asked relaxed, casual questions about my hobbies, career goals and how I would make a positive impact if I was crowned Miss Ireland. The relief among my fellow contestants once the interview section was over was palpable, and after a bite of lunch, we went upstairs to the hair and make-up suite to get ready for the competition that evening – although I felt more comfortable doing my own make-up, as I just wanted to look like myself. Later that night, as I walked the catwalk for the first time, my whole chin trembled with nerves and I was convinced that everybody in the room could see it. I managed to relax after that and began to enjoy it, as we all had a bit of fun chatting backstage. I can still recall the pumping music, flashing lights and wild cheers from my family and friends in the crowd when my name was announced as the winner. It felt surreal, like an out-of-body experience, as the custom-made Newbridge Silverware tiara was placed on my head and the winner's sash draped across my evening gown. Heart thumping, I posed for photos as my parents rushed over to hug me, and the celebrations continued long into the night.

I had really enjoyed my first year in college, especially the social side of life. I joined various societies, played netball for UCD and made the most of the campus facilities. Yet when winning Miss Ireland automatically put me forward for the Miss World competition to be held in December of that year, I knew that I'd have to defer. Miss World is a huge international competition and the contract stipulated that if you won, you had to be prepared to commit to a year of work to fulfil your Miss World obligations.

I can't imagine that my tutors in UCD were used to being asked for a deferral to enter a beauty competition, but they were very supportive, and I'd surprised myself by really enjoying my time as Miss Ireland. I'd been very busy since my win with TV appearances and fashion shows as well as a lot of charity work, which I loved. As you can imagine, it was a whole new world for a nineteen-year-old. I felt that this novel adventure would only ever be temporary so I threw myself into it, travelling all over the country for events, meeting lots of new people, doing photoshoots, having my hair and make-up done by professionals. I never expected to come away from it as Miss World.

Once we had gathered in China, I soon realised that many of the contestants took the competition a great deal more seriously than I did. For many of them, winning Miss World could be a ticket out of a poorer country or would give them a whole new platform. In fact, I remember one girl who had a huge manual that she used to consult, full of instructions about etiquette and outfits. I quickly learned that I was not in the competition to make lifelong friends!

The preparation for the month in China had been pretty demanding. I packed about four giant suitcases with all of the outfits I'd need for the various events, and I quickly realised that I wouldn't be able to manage it all by myself. A fantastic lady called Lisa Fitzpatrick came over to the house to style me and help me to pack. She was very organised, writing out a list of what I'd need and for which occasion and even arranged for me to borrow some dresses and other outfits. Sometimes, I would need three outfits a day: if we were filming in the morning, we might need a dress, trouser suit or skirt suit, then in the afternoon a cocktail dress, and if there was a gala dinner, I'd need an evening gown complete with clutch bag and jewellery.

Many people have preconceptions about beauty pageants, and I was exactly the same before I took part, but I told myself that, whatever happened, I would embrace it as a new experience. I'd never been to China, so I was excited about exploring a new country. The final competition was to be held in Sanya, but before that, we had a month of touring around the country and it was fascinating. We started off in Hong Kong, which was vast, brimming with energy and bustling with activity, and a melting pot of different nationalities. Secondly, we went on to Shanghai, which was impressive. It feels quite western in many ways, with the colonial buildings on the Bund facing the river, which looks amazing when it's lit up. I also remember Xi'an, home to the Terracotta Army, and Guangzhou, which was one of the biggest cities I'd ever seen, home to more than forty-six million people. Wherever we went we were mobbed because this was the first time the competition had been held in China and there was a huge buzz about it. The purpose-built Crown of Beauty theatre was designed especially for the final competition, which was in the 'Hawaii of China' on Hainan, one of the islands off the coast of mainland China, with its almost tropical climate, holiday resorts and beautiful beaches.

Once I had worked out the logistics, I began to really enjoy myself. It's intimidating and overwhelming to find yourself in a competition like Miss World, but it's full of new experiences and I had fun. It shattered my preconceptions about beauty pageants: none of these girls were airheads. They were professionals or undergraduates and ambitious, driven women who were taking unpaid time out of their normal lives, as I was, to enhance their life experience, to gain a platform in their own country or to raise awareness of charity issues. I might not have gone there thinking that I'd take it seriously, but I quickly adapted. The atmosphere was very competitive, so I had to tap into my competitive side. I certainly do have one!

Sometimes, this could get quite funny. The minute a photographer showed up, elbows would be sharpened and we'd all try to push our way to the front, or if the photo involved babies or children, they would be grabbed for the photo. I quickly learned to anticipate the rush to make it into the centre of every picture, complete with my biggest, cheesiest smile. But even though it was highly competitive, it wasn't bitchy or unpleasant: it was just a professional job for many of the women there – and they were all there to win.

A lot of people ask me about the bikini aspect of the Miss World competition and how I felt about it. I'm not sure what the situation is nowadays, but back then Julia Morley, the competition organiser, was very protective. I remember her saying, 'I don't want you girls going onstage in high heels and a bikini. It's not appropriate. If we are doing a bikini section, I want you barefoot on the beach, as you would usually be when wearing a bikini.' She was determined that it wouldn't look tacky in any way. And while the atmosphere in the stadium was pretty intense, it was all very elegant. There was also a number of fast-track competitions that encouraged us to showcase our abilities. Apart from the bikini one, which I was pleasantly surprised to win, there was a sports competition, one to reward charity work and a talent competition. I wrote a poem for it about my experience in China, and some of the girls had impressive talent in music and dance.

We were split into groups of six and had a chaperone, who apparently reported to the organisation on our conduct. It didn't bother me because Miss World ultimately want a brand ambassador, a representative who can be trusted to speak to the media, to dress and behave appropriately, so I wanted to make a good impression. I was aware that I always had to act professionally, no matter what I was doing; and we were doing a lot. The TV audience only sees the more commercial side of the competition, but we also did a lot of filming, press conferences, dinners with heads of state and visits to hospitals and orphanages. It was great fun and really educational, if exhausting.

I'll never forget the night I won Miss World and, without a doubt, it changed my life. Winning the bikini section had fast-tracked me into the top twenty finalists, and I was thrilled with that, so when my name was called out as a top five finalist alongside the representatives from Canada, China, India and the Philippines, I almost froze in shock. Just as in the Miss Ireland competition, we were asked a question on stage and judge Jackie Chan asked me what I felt my best qualities are. I answered that I'm a woman of loyalty, integrity and honesty and that being crowned Miss World would give me a voice to support and represent women internationally. We weren't given our questions in advance and I remember wondering if what I had just said made any sense at all. The surging adrenaline in my system had caused my head to go blank and I'm sure the other girls felt the same. After all, the event organisers estimated the global audience to be around two billion people.

My heart was thumping as Julia Morley began to read out the names of the runners-up, starting with Miss China, Guan Qi, and Miss Canada, Nazanin Afshin-Jam. As I heard the sentence 'And the winner is ... Miss Ireland' ring out across the packed theatre, I searched for my parents' faces in the crowd. They were jumping up and down, screaming and waving at me. I simply couldn't believe it. The rest was a blur as I walked shakily across to the winner's throne to be crowned by Miss World 2002, Azra Akin, and then proceeded to do the 'lap of honour' we had all practised during rehearsals, waving to the cheering crowd. Later that night, I sat at the head table at the final gala dinner of the Miss World 2003 competition, and as I was invited onstage to make my acceptance speech, I remember feeling faint from what was the most exhilarating, exhausting and exciting day of my life. Spotting me wobbling, Mum and Dad brought me upstairs after the main course to relax and I fell fast asleep on the sofa in their hotel room, my Miss World sash still wrapped around me. Waking up the next morning, the events of the night before felt like a wild, vivid dream. Did that all really happen? I still find it hard to believe that I was once Miss World, and someday I'll tell my children all about it.

I recently came across a clip of me appearing on the *Late Late Show* with Pat Kenny, after I'd won Miss World, and he asked me if I was aware of the excitement back in Ireland. I wasn't, but I was so thrilled that everyone at home had enjoyed it. Irish people are fantastic at getting behind someone and really cheering them on, and when I returned to all the press clippings that Mum and Dad had kept for me, I was really touched. I did know that I was the bookies' favourite for the few days leading up to the final, but I had tried not to dwell on it. Dad said to me, 'Don't pay any attention, it's just speculation,' and he was right. I had done my best and had represented myself and my country as best I could. The rest was just noise, if you like.

I wasn't naïve – I did realise that beauty sells – but before the era of social media, there wasn't nearly as much scrutiny of women, their bodies, their hair, their clothes. I find that an interesting development because I use social media as a tool myself, so I'm aware of the pros and cons and the fact that, if you are a public face, it's better for your mental health to pay little or no attention to negativity and trolling. Fortunately, the majority of the comments I've received over the years have been positive. And when I talked about my fertility issues, people were overwhelmingly kind and supportive. When used in a positive and beneficial way, social media is an effective means to connect with others, promote businesses and stay in contact with family and friends. I can't stand the negativity and bullying that, all too often, come with it, and while I don't experience much trolling, I use the block button if I do rather than getting involved, and I don't tend to read direct messages from people I don't know because a hateful message can ruin your day if you're feeling particularly sensitive or vulnerable.

The opinion of a person who doesn't know me and hasn't lived a second of my life doesn't bother me in the slightest, but it's the idea that they would take time out of their day to spew negativity at a stranger that shocks me most. I like Instagram but I take it with a pinch of salt too and don't allow myself to either believe everything I see or compare myself to others – I think that's an important lesson to learn and to keep in mind. Enjoy it but draw a line between social media and reality and don't allow it to take over your life or get in the way of real events, human face-to-face contact and relationships.

I must admit that I worry about how I will navigate the world of social media with Sophia, Hugo and Oscar when they're older and start to show an interest in it. We don't know how it will evolve over the next decade or so, and if it remains as dominant as it is now, then I just hope that I can safely guide my children through it and teach them not to waste their precious time worrying about what people think or say on it. They're nothing more than strangers seeing curated snapshots of your life, generally without context or understanding of your thought processes, challenges, insecurities, priorities or lifestyle. There's simply no way you can fully understand another person's perspective without living their life and that's why I believe it's so important to be non-judgemental, open-minded and empathetic towards others. Nobody should feel the need to explain themselves or reveal the more difficult parts of life, but as I have discovered through sharing details of our fertility struggles online, others can appreciate you showing and discussing your vulnerabilities. Acknowledging that life isn't perfect shows you are human and normal, and almost everybody can relate to feeling scared, anxious or insecure at some stage in their life. None of us gets through life without our fair share of challenges, and I feel that it's important to recognise that.

In May 2021 I shared an image on Instagram of the bruises I'd developed from injecting myself with heparin for nine months during 2020 due to my inherited Factor V Leiden thrombophilia, and it was eye-opening to discover there are many more women like me who also had to inject themselves to help sustain a pregnancy. Discussing these obstacles in life can help to raise awareness and make others feel less alone. Ultimately, it's human connection and all of the positive associated emotions that makes life fulfilling and meaningful.

On 6 December 2003, I was very proud to represent Ireland while wearing my hot-pink custom-made evening gown by Irish designer Cathy de Stafford. The following year, 2004, passed in a blur of Miss World travel, promotion and charity work, and for someone who had been a student up to a few months before, it was a new and exciting pace of life. I can still remember Addis Ababa, the capital of Ethiopia, because it was fascinating, so rich in culture and history and with such lovely people. Then I'd pop over to Beijing for the weekend to walk for a designer in Beijing Fashion Week; the next, I'd be Grand Marshal of the St Patrick's Day parade in Toronto or making a TV appearance in the UK or Germany. The following weekend I'd be flying to Chicago for an event and then on to Des Moines, Iowa to co-present a twenty-four-hour charity telethon. At times, my head would spin, but you have the energy for it when you're nineteen. I quickly learned to embrace it all because it was only for a year, after which my life would return to normal, or so I thought.

I returned to college in September 2004 and from then until December I combined my studies with my Miss World obligations. I remember staying in a Hong Kong hotel overlooking Victoria Harbour and writing an essay on the architectural characteristics of Gothic cathedrals for my history of art module. Somehow, I managed to blend the two relatively smoothly for another few months before I handed over my crown to the 2004 Miss World winner and concentrated on my final two years in university. In early 2005, I signed a contract to be brand ambassador for a popular European travelling ice show called Holiday on Ice. From the beginning of that year, I'd go into college to attend a morning lecture or tutorial, then catch a plane to Germany, Paris or Amsterdam to do a photo shoot, film a TV advert or walk the red carpet of a premiere, then return to Dublin the next morning and pop into college for my afternoon lecture. It was intense, but I've always thrived on being busy and having a variety of interests. Despite the gruelling schedule, I still managed to make time to meet up with friends and I never missed birthday celebrations and other important family occasions. Anyone close to me was always very supportive of my choices and it became a normal way of life. I was constantly packing and unpacking suitcases!

Part of the reason I was able to juggle the two roles was because I've always been pretty focused. Once I set my mind on a goal, I apply myself fully until I achieve it. This has turned out to be a useful skill over the past few years, though I'd be the first to admit that that drive makes it hard for me to relax. I'd enjoyed college in first year, hanging out in the student bar, having drinks at lunchtime. I considered blue alcopops and a bag of chips to be a solid meal as a student. But I was much more focused in third year, probably because I was keen to just get my degree. Wherever I went in the world, I would bring my books and laptop with me; I'd often be in the back of a car on my way to an event with my college books on my knee. I was delighted to sit the last exam of my UCD finals in May 2006, but then I really had to make a decision, as so many of us do at that age. It reminded me a bit of the film *Sliding Doors*, where each door will take you in a very different direction. I had to work out what kind of person I was.

Plenty of interesting opportunities were arising in my new Miss World life. I'd signed up with a London modelling agency called Storm and travelled regularly between London and Germany for work. On the other hand, I had worked hard enough in my final sociology exams to achieve a first-class honours degree and, as a result, I was offered a scholarship to study for a PhD in sociological research. I loved the idea of getting a doctorate and being Dr Davison! However, I realised that perhaps I wanted to do it for the title, rather than to make an impact in the academic field. I had really enjoyed sociology, but I knew that it wasn't my passion. I also felt that I'd focused extremely hard for months studying for my finals and now was the time to work, travel and explore the opportunities available to me. So that's what I did. It never even entered my mind that I'd still be working in this business eighteen years later and that it would be my career.

I'll quite happily admit to liking being in control of things. Who doesn't? Everyone wants to think that they are master of their own fate; that they can shape their future in exactly the way they want to. However, if the last few years have taught me anything, it's that no amount of control will make your every wish come true. You can't have everything just because you want it, no matter how badly. It was a tough lesson for me to learn, but a humbling one.

CHAPTER 2

LOVE AND LOSS

How many of us think that pregnancy is a natural process? Most people, I'd imagine. Before Wes and I had difficulties, I naïvely believed that pregnancies usually have a successful outcome and, depending on their life situations, people are thrilled to expand their families or worried about how they'd cope with the various emotional, physical and financial challenges of parenthood. We were married at the age of thirty and I had planned to have our first baby at thirty-two, our second at thirty-four and perhaps a third a couple of years after that, if we were lucky enough.

My mum had had a long fertility struggle before she conceived me under what her doctor considered to be miraculous circumstances. She had suffered multiple miscarriages and a life-threatening ectopic pregnancy. She was rushed to hospital in a collapsed state and her obstetrician managed to remove the foetus from her burst fallopian tube while retaining the tube. Some months later, her obstetrician, who had recently qualified in micro-surgery in London, operated. He did his best to repair the tube where the ectopic pregnancy had occurred and had to remove the other tube, which was blocked. Mum was told that her chances of conceiving were extremely slim and that a subsequent pregnancy could again be ectopic. Luckily, and thanks to the skill and foresight of her obstetrician, she conceived all three of her babies through the tube that had been badly damaged by the ectopic pregnancy.

Despite being aware of my mum's difficulties, infertility and miscarriage weren't really on my radar. A couple of close friends had experienced miscarriages, but subsequently had successful full-term pregnancies. Apart from that, pregnancy loss just wasn't discussed. I had no idea that statistically one in six confirmed pregnancies ends in miscarriage. Why is it so shrouded in mystery? And why did I feel so ashamed and guilty when it happened to us? I'm grateful every day that Wes and I agreed about every procedure and fully supported each other, as fertility issues and miscarriage can put a serious strain on relationships.

I first met Wes in the summer of 2006. I had recently completed my UCD finals and was having a dance in a local nightclub when I bumped into him. The memory is a bit hazy now, as I was with some girlfriends and he was with another group, so I said 'hi' just in passing. A couple of months later, he sent me a message on Bebo. Millennials might not remember this early social networking site, but we loved it. Looking back, I don't think it even counted as social media – just a personalised internet page with your likes and dis-likes, top friends, a snazzy wallpaper and plenty of unfiltered photos from nights out. It was all harmless and fun.

I had uploaded some pictures from a family holiday to Mauritius during Christmas and New Year and Wes had sent me a message about how much he'd enjoyed his first time at the sister resort with his family the previous year, so we got chatting – virtually, that is. Back in the mid-noughties, meeting and speaking to strangers on the internet was con-sidered risky, and my friends were understandably concerned. They warned me to be careful, which amuses us now. It was all very innocent chat about our pets, our families and where we lived. We ended up having plenty in common, and after about a month of chatting online every evening, Wes ever-so-casually mentioned the opening party for a local bar. 'Look, I'm going with my friends, are you thinking of going?'

'Well,' I replied, equally casually, 'I'll see if I can gather a few friends together – maybe see you there.' I went with three of my girlfriends and he arrived with three of his guy pals and it was very relaxed, with a late-night group trip to pick up a burger and chips on the way home. He seemed like a friendly, fun and relaxed kind of guy. I was especially impressed with how happy he was to sit down at the table with my friends when he arrived and that he remembered all of their names later on in the night! We got on very well and spent much of the night just laughing together, telling funny stories and dancing with the others.

After that first evening out together, I flew to New York for a week-long holiday with friends and he went on a trip to Florida so I didn't see him for a couple of weeks, although plenty of text messages were exchanged. Our first 'official' date was in September 2006, and that time we opted for a movie. I think the cinema is a great icebreaker on a date early in a relationship because if you don't have much in common, you can just focus on the film. But as it happened, Wes and I didn't stop chatting. I felt really relaxed with him and there was a lovely natural feel to our time spent together. Also, beginning our relationship on Bebo gave us a good story to tell, at a time when meeting online was a bit of a novelty. There was no swiping right in 2006 and selfies certainly didn't exist!

Wes was busy working in the family business and he was very laid-back about my career. Still, I don't think he was ready for the attention that our relationship initially attracted. The first time we attended an event together, we were photographed and there was a bit of interest from the gossip columnists in my new man. I had become used to working with the media during my Miss World year, and it was an aspect of my job that had also become a part of my everyday life. Wes subsequently became a lot more private and he prefers to stay out of the limelight, also keeping a fairly low profile on social media. I respect that he's a private person and doesn't benefit from being in the public eye. He has his business to run and his own life to lead, which is not online.

With the advent of social media, it's become harder to separate public and private life, but I've always preferred to keep a little distance between my personal and professional lives. Wes and I attend events together occasionally, but at home we like to have our own happy, private family life. For that reason, you won't see our whole house or our children directly photographed online. Wes is very aware of maintaining privacy and security. He feels strongly that he doesn't want our children's faces on the internet and I agree. It's a personal choice and we would never judge anyone else's decisions, but we feel that children don't have a choice in the matter and that it's our responsibility as parents to keep them safe until they're old enough to make up their own minds about their online presence. Nobody needs to know what they look like, apart from family and friends. The internet can be a dark and dangerous place, as we all know.

This might seem somewhat contradictory, since I'm writing a book detailing our fertility journey, but we both strongly feel that it's important to share our personal story in the hope of giving others some comfort, reassurance and inspiration.

It's important to document all the detail and even though some of the memories might not be happy ones, they are very much part of our experience and therefore need to be acknowledged. As we discovered, the road to parenthood can be incredibly complex and circuitous, with no guarantee of a successful outcome. Infertility and baby loss, no matter what stage of pregnancy a woman is at, can be a profoundly lonely, devastating and traumatic experience for both an individual and a couple. We realise that there's no 'correct' way of dealing with the intense emotions and desperate sense of loss, but speaking in confidence to close friends or family members and sharing human experiences can be deeply cathartic.

Above the sofa in the living room, there's a huge photo of Wes and me on our wedding day in 2014. I often look at it, reminiscing about how happy we were to celebrate the next chapter in our lives together. We had our whole future ahead of us. There was something so exhilarating about that feeling, wondering where we'd travel to, the family we'd create and the adventures we'd have together.

We had been together for seven and a half years when he proposed to me on the beach in Mauritius on Sunday 6 January 2013 during a Christmas-holiday break with my family. We had gone out for a late-morning walk down the beach, as we always did, hand in hand, just chatting about the beautiful view across the lagoon to the mountains beyond. I remember thinking that he seemed subdued, and as we reached the furthest point of the beach, he turned to face me and disappeared downwards. For a split second, I thought he had collapsed from the heat! But out from the pocket of his combat shorts emerged a ring box, with a diamond ring sparkling in the sunshine. We both broke down in tears, hugging and kissing, as he asked me to marry him.

We ran back to my family, tears still rolling down our cheeks and screeching in excitement as we told them our news and I showed them my new engagement ring. What a moment! Granny had come away with us, and she gave us a huge hug, grinning in delight. We celebrated with a long lunch on the beach and many fellow hotel guests came over to congratulate us. We've dubbed the day 'Champagne Sunday'!

We waited a year and a half to get married, as I was keen to focus on my nutritional therapy course and take our time to make plans with the guidance and advice of our wonderful wedding planner, Tara Fay. We chose to have a humanist wedding in the Merrion Hotel, Dublin on 16 May 2014, with just our immediate families and the bridal party attending the ceremony and celebratory lunch afterwards. It was a beautiful, intimate day and the sun shone brightly all afternoon as we sat outside in the hotel's elegant garden. A fortnight later, on 1 June 2014, we enjoyed a bigger celebration with our families and friends in a pretty boutique hotel called Atzaró Agroturismo, in the heart of Ibiza. The estate's beautifully manicured gardens, with orange grove, palm trees, pools and pavilions, made a stunning setting for our special day.

As I mentioned earlier, having a family was very much part of our plans. It seemed like a natural next step in our relationship and one for which we felt ready. Six years ago, we embarked on a mission that we assumed would be easy. When Wes and I had met at twenty-two, becoming parents seemed a long way in the future. He has two sisters and a brother and I'm very close to my two brothers, so we both loved the idea of a busy, happy family home. I didn't feel particularly maternal at that age, though, as I was focused on building my career, studying and writing and releasing my two plant-based cookbooks, *Eat Yourself Beautiful* and *Eat Yourself Fit* with Gill Books. It was over a year into our marriage before we began to think seriously about the prospect of babies.

We were ecstatic when I got pregnant straight away. It was early 2016 and I woke up one morning feeling a bit different. I remember so clearly being out for a walk with friends and thinking that I didn't feel well. I was lightheaded, tired and slightly queasy – a little bit lower in energy, perhaps. I didn't say a word to Wes but spent the whole day thinking about it, wondering whether to chance a trip to the local pharmacy for a pregnancy test or if it might be too early. Eventually, curiosity prevailed, and I'll never forget staring in wide-eyed amazement and disbelief as the two pink lines on the test confirmed what I already suspected. I was four and a half weeks pregnant. My first thought was that I couldn't believe it had happened so quickly, and my second was how would we manage? I expect that any newly pregnant woman feels the same way, with that heady mixture of excitement and anxiety about the future.

I waited until Wes arrived home from work that day to tell him the news by casually handing him a small container and asking him to take a look inside. I had popped the positive test inside a long, narrow jewellery box and managed to record his shocked expression when he opened it up and realised what he was looking at. I can still see the look of surprise and excitement on his face, mixed with all of the other emotions that emerge with finding out that you're going to be a dad. We both broke down in elated tears at the idea of becoming first-time parents later that year. In the depths of our fertility struggles, I sometimes looked back at that video, both cringing at our innocence and wishing it hadn't been so ruthlessly torn from us.

Meanwhile, I was anxious to tell my family. I'm very close to my mum and dad and I couldn't wait to share our news with them. I knew they'd be delighted at the idea of becoming grandparents for the first time. We drove down to my family home in Co. Wicklow for lunch with my parents and brothers, as we frequently do, but this time we were bursting to tell them our news. I barely said a word through lunch, letting the conversation flow around me while I nibbled on my food and ignored my glass of wine. Eventually, I blurted,

'We have something tell you,' in the middle of a chat about the weather. 'I'm pregnant!' I said, tears welling up. There were hugs and kisses and cheers from my two brothers and lots of excited questions about the due date and how I was feeling. I basked in the pure joy of our announcement. At just under five weeks pregnant, my secret was out.

I thought about my due date in autumn 2016 and how I would tell my friends when the time was right. I couldn't wait to chat to them about motherhood, make lists of what to buy for our baby and begin to think about nursery decor. I daydreamed about names and how we'd spend our first Christmas with our new son or daughter. We had so much to look forward to. Some of my best friends had already given birth to their first or even second babies at that stage, and I'd watched their bumps grow and their newborns arrive and joined in the excitement of baby showers and shopping for gifts. I thought that's what happened in all pregnancies. So when Mum pulled me aside to sound a note of caution, I thought she was fussing too much. 'Be careful because things can go wrong at this early stage, Rosie,' she said. I appreciated her advice and knew that she wasn't trying to puncture my excitement, but in my naivety, I believed that two healthy young people would have no problems at all.

Over the next couple of weeks, I took more pregnancy tests to check and double-check that I was still pregnant, watching with delight as the lines in the little window grew darker. There's something so primal and exhilarating about a life growing inside you, and the slight vertigo combined with increasing nausea and a heightened sense of smell gave me a thrill. Every little hormone surge and new symptom was a sign that my pregnancy was progressing. My GP confirmed my pregnancy at five and a half weeks and suggested I make an appointment for my first early pregnancy scan. I booked an eight-week ultrasound, excitedly counting down the days to my appointment at the National Maternity Hospital in Holles Street, when Wes and I hoped to see the flicker of a healthy foetal heartbeat.

When you become pregnant for the first time, you cross over into the world of the prospective parent and you begin to view life differently. You start to imagine how it might feel to be a family of three, what your relationship will be like with your baby, whether you'll be a good mum or dad and whether you'll be able to provide for this little person, nurturing and protecting them as they grow from baby to child and beyond. It's daunting and wildly exciting at the same time. Back then, it all seemed so easy and straightforward to just get pregnant and have a baby. We were young, fit and healthy, what could possibly go wrong?

I first realised that something was wrong at six weeks pregnant. I woke up one Sunday morning and I felt a bit different, a little less nauseated, tired and bloated. I tried to reassure myself that I'd probably just had a better night's sleep, although I couldn't shake that creeping feeling of dread. Then, a couple of days later, the spotting started. In a panic, I rang my GP, Dr Penny Bleakley, who was calm and reassuring. She told me that spotting can happen in early pregnancy and often it's nothing to worry about. She advised me to relax and let her know if it became any heavier. For the next forty-eight hours, I did my best to distract myself, even though I could hardly think about anything else. The blood disappeared for a day or so and then returned. Wes and I were both on tenterhooks.

On the following Wednesday night, as we were getting ready for bed, I had a sudden feeling that something was very wrong. I can't fully explain it, but something in me knew that I was losing the pregnancy. Maybe those of you who have gone through the experience will understand. Perhaps it's just hindsight making me think this, I'm not sure. It was as if I could feel those pregnancy hormones finally draining out of my body.

I was in the bathroom when the intense, excruciating cramping started. It was like nothing I'd experienced before. Calling for Wes, I slumped onto the bathroom tiles and began to cry. In between the breathless sobs, I remember repeatedly apologising to him that I had failed to keep our baby alive, that my body had let us down and destroyed our dream of having a family. Soon after I broke into a sweat, lying on the floor writhing because the pain was that intense. It seemed as if I was losing an ocean of blood, too. Poor Wes had no idea how to help and, quite honestly, there was nothing for him to do. At that stage I didn't feel capable of even standing up to get into the car and be driven to hospital. All I wanted to do was curl up in a ball on the floor. I eventually urged him to go back to bed, so one of us at least could get some rest, then I sat and cried my heart out. Your whole idea of the world comes crashing down when you start having a miscarriage. Along with the discomfort and the bleeding come the endless questions. Was it that cup of coffee I drank? Should I not have gone for that walk? Is my reproductive system in some way dysfunctional? That's where the destructive pattern of self-blame began for me.

I was desperate to ring Mum, but I didn't want to wake her in the middle of the night, so I fumbled for my phone and called my brother Michael, who was in Los Angeles at the time. Because of the eight-hour time difference, I didn't feel quite so bad disturbing him. I blubbed at him, 'I'm lying on the floor having a miscarriage. I just need someone to talk to.' He was very sweet and concerned for me, which was just what I needed. I was probably trying to protect Wes at that point from the grief, yet I felt such an overwhelming desire to tell someone and to share what was going on. My brother's support was fantastic. This might seem strange to some, but we were brought up to talk to trusted family and friends and not to bottle things up, which is a lesson I've really taken to heart. I've always been very open to sharing and listening to other people's problems. Telling Michael didn't worry me at all because I knew how kind and supportive he'd be.

After a couple of hours, the pain thankfully stopped and I managed to drag myself to bed. I fell into a deep, exhausted sleep. The following morning, I rang the hospital to tell them and I was asked to go in for a scan to check that I'd had a full miscarriage. If you've had a miscarriage, you'll know about the painful and difficult aftermath. Far from a miracle of nature, it's an intensely physical process of loss. Depending on the stage of pregnancy you reached, there's generally a lot of blood loss, clots and tissue to pass. I always had 'complete' miscarriages, but friends of mine have had procedures called a dilation and curettage (D&C) to surgically remove pregnancy tissue in the uterus. I count myself lucky that I never required one. But despite that, a miscarriage at any stage is the end of a pregnancy and the end of a dream. From the moment you cast your eyes across that positive pregnancy test, you calculate your due date and begin to imagine cradling a newborn baby in your arms. For me, pregnancy loss came as a huge shock. That something so precious can be ripped from you so suddenly is deeply traumatic. Miscarriage steals your innocence about pregnancy – that it's all a natural process of growth and love – and for me, it's never been quite the same since. Friends of mine who have had miscarriages and gone on to have healthy babies agree with me that, no matter how happy the outcome, there is always a little part of you that remembers that awful time.

It took me a considerable length of time to recover from that first experience, both physically and emotionally. The sudden and devastating physical loss of it really slowed me down. One day we were excitedly planning our future as a family of three and just weeks later it was all taken from us. It took me ages to work through and understand the psychological impact of miscarriage for both partners. Overall, it made me appreciate how precious and fragile life can be.

That is when it began to dawn on me what a mystery pregnancy actually is. We can do so much medically nowadays, but much of diagnosing and treating fertility problems remains a grey area. For example, I've always found IVF an amazing process – being able to implant an embryo into a womb via a tiny tube – but it came as quite a shock to me that, in my own case, the answers to my problems would be a lot harder to find.

My doctor had reassured me that miscarriages are more common than I thought and I'd probably go on to have a perfectly normal and healthy full-term pregnancy. We waited, we recovered and then we tried again. And I got pregnant again. I was thrilled, of course, but this time I was more cautious. I decided to wait before telling anybody apart from Wes and my mum. I was so hopeful and just wanted to be sure that this second pregnancy would last.

I booked in to the hospital at about five weeks pregnant for a blood test to ensure that my hCG level – the pregnancy hormone – was rising as it should be in early pregnancy. The nurse who took my blood was gently reassuring, talking to me about all kinds of things to keep my mind off the test and I began to relax, feeling more positive. But when I got the call some hours later to tell me that my levels were too low and this pregnancy was going to fail, it felt as if I had failed too. My heart sank as I slowly walked to my car to go home and tell Wes and Mum that my second pregnancy was doomed. I was less shocked this time, because the first miscarriage had given me an insight into dealing with the trauma of pregnancy loss, but I was still devastated.

We allowed ourselves some time to recover and rebuild our strength, and I became more determined. *This isn't going to get the better of me*, I thought. *We're going to keep trying. And we're going to succeed.*

The other aspect that startled me, but probably won't surprise those of you who have experienced more than one miscarriage, is that until you have suffered three of them nothing is really investigated. Our consultant obstetrician told us that it was my body's way of rejecting a foetus that wasn't going to develop, most likely due to a genetic anomaly, and we simply had to try again when we felt ready to – although he recommended waiting a full cycle. But losing that primal feeling of pregnancy, where every cell in your body is directed towards growing this new life inside you, was very hard to cope with. That sense of shared excitement, of hope in the future, is gone. And your plans suddenly change, too. From thinking about the world from the perspective of a parent to be, you're suddenly back to the world as it always has been.

I had fourteen early miscarriages between 2016 and 2018. Each followed the same pattern of an initial positive home pregnancy test, only for hormone levels to fade and disappear by about six weeks. My heart sank every time the pregnancy failed and the inevitable bleeding began. I felt that I was failing too but we never lost that little flicker of hope. No matter what you're put through, and the barriers you face, you think, just one more cycle – let's just try again. You try not to get too technical about things, despite your forensic awareness of when you might be ovulating and what stage your cycle is at. In my experience, trying for a baby for as long as we did takes the romance right out of it. It undoubtedly put pressure on us as a couple, and it can be a fairly tedious experience when you're both worn out after a long day at work. The idea of missing out on that crucial window of opportunity each month terrified me. I can still remember ringing Wes in a panic one afternoon when I realised I was ovulating, insisting he come home from work immediately, while ushering my mother, who was visiting, out the door!

With each subsequent early miscarriage, I felt the loss, but there was also a growing sense of frustration at what I saw as my inability to stay pregnant. Despite being well aware that fertility problems can be due to the man or the woman, I repeatedly blamed myself, believing that I was defective in some way. There was something about me that just didn't work properly. That my body was broken.

It was only after our third miscarriage that the doctor said, 'OK, it's time to do some tests.' Wes and I were relieved – at last, we thought, we might find some answers to the mystery. The tests were certainly comprehensive. We took the following tests between 2016 and 2017:

- A hormone profile to check levels of progesterone and FSH, or follicle stimulating hormone
- A thrombophilia screen, which tests for inherited or predisposed deficiencies in blood clotting
- A blood test to check levels of TSH, or thyroid-stimulating hormone
- Karyotyping for both of us to check for chromosomal abnormalities
- Semen analysis in Wes's case
- A homocysteine assay to check for deficiencies in B12 or folate that might affect the pregnancy
- An AMH, or anti-Müllerian hormone, test, which can indicate ovarian reserve
- Infectious diseases tests
- MTHFR mutation test – this might sound like a swear word, but it actually refers to a genetic mutation that can cause a number of health problems and might have a role in miscarriage
- Tests for levels of folic acid, iron and vitamin B12

- A thromboelastogram, which tests again for blood coagulation
- A test for prolactin, a hormone that is produced by your pituitary gland that can have a role in infertility
- Tests for anti-thyroid antibodies and antiphospholipid antibodies, both present in autoimmune diseases thought to play a possible role in infertility

A little overwhelming, isn't it? I've listed them here because I want to show that infertility is an incredibly complex issue, the causes of which can vary so much from couple to couple. And sometimes, after all of that, the actual cause of infertility remains a mystery. In my case, when the test results came back everything was clear apart from the diagnosis of an inherited genetic mutation called Heterozygous Factor V Leiden, which is present on Mum's side of the family. It means that my blood has an increased tendency to form abnormal blood clots that can potentially block blood vessels. As a result, I was prescribed daily anticoagulant injections plus low-dose aspirin for future pregnancies. My doctor wasn't entirely sure that that was what lay behind the failed pregnancies, but it was decided that it might help and I agreed. If he'd told me to enter the 100-metre sprint in the Olympics against Usain Bolt, I'd have agreed! When you are desperate to have a baby and a solution seems to present itself, you'll do anything. A nurse explained to me how best to administer the heparin and I was sent home with a yellow bin to dispose of the used needles. At the time, the idea of self-injecting daily seemed daunting, but I remember feeling hopeful that it would help me to hold onto my next pregnancy. Little did I know how many more injections I'd have.

I'm also a serial problem-solver by nature, so I took the initiative by doing my own research, asking a lot of my own questions and even suggesting tests, supported by my GP and by Wes. I'd advise anyone going through fertility issues to ask questions and suggest areas that might not already have been investigated. I was curious about what was happening and always interested in looking at every angle and possibility. My studies had helped me to develop my research skills, to read data with confidence and to ask the right questions. I was proactive about making appointments with fertility clinics and researching specialists, a process that was exhausting, but one that we both felt was worth it.

By April 2017, the fertility doctor that I had been seeing was running out of ideas and decided to refer me to a second specialist to have a hysteroscopy. As he explained, 'This involves taking a look at the inside of the womb to see if there are any structural issues with it.' I thought that it sounded quite promising and perhaps my uterus was the problem. Full of hope, I was booked into hospital for the procedure, which is conducted under general anaesthetic. Once the doctor had investigated my womb lining with a tiny camera, he proceeded to cut out a 'septum' at the fundus – or top – of my uterus. It was small, taking up approximately ten per cent of my womb. The tissue of a uterine septum is fibrous, rather than spongy, so it can reduce the likelihood of normal implantation. He also did what's called a uterine, or endometrial, scratch under anaesthetic. Theoretically, what this does is disturb the lining of the womb to encourage it to repair the area of the scratch and to release certain hormones and chemicals to support embryo implantation. Finally, the doctor did a swab to check for any bacterial overgrowth around the cervix and nothing showed up.

I had some discomfort for a few days following the procedure, and we were advised to wait a cycle or two before trying to conceive again. By June 2017, I was pregnant. Wes and I were both so happy – surely, this time it would work. I had convinced myself that the septum had been the root cause of our issues and removing it was the solution. But of course, at the six-week mark, the pregnancy failed again. I lost hope at that point and found myself slipping into that dark place of despair. *Why can't we establish what's wrong with me?* I thought. *Maybe it's time to give up.* I was exhausted, not only by the losses, but also by the constant invasions that come with infertility: all the blood tests, the procedures and the interventions. After spending a number of days seriously considering my role and future as a woman and a wife, I found myself urging Wes to consider leaving me to find a partner to have a family with, assuring him that

I'd be supportive and understanding. As a woman, I knew that I could offer more to the world than just my ability – or inability – to procreate, but as his wife, I felt an enormous weight of responsibility and guilt. Wes and I had got married in the hopes of having a family and I had started to convince myself that I was getting in the way of his dreams and it would be kinder to set him free.

By that stage, he had taken all the fertility tests recommended for the male partner and they hadn't shown any irregularities, so we knew the problem lay with me. His sister had two children at this point and I could see how much he loved being an uncle, yet I couldn't seem to make him a dad. Thankfully, he told me firmly that leaving me was not an option. We laugh now, but at the time I was serious. I couldn't keep dragging him along this distressing rollercoaster of pregnancy and loss when he wanted so badly to become a father. I felt that it wasn't fair, and if he could achieve his dreams with someone else, I would support him even though it would break my heart. It seems like madness now, but fertility struggles can bring you to a very dark emotional place. Now, I understand that Wes was going through it with me and was every bit as upset as I was with each miscarriage, but he felt that his role was to support me, not to examine his own feelings. Yet partners are losing the baby too. Their dreams are being crushed as well, but they're expected to be strong and supportive. Wes knew he had to hold me up, so he couldn't crumble. When

I had that conversation with him, urging him to move on, he said, 'Rosie, it's you I want to have a family with, and if it doesn't happen, we'll figure it out.'

The irony was that, while all of this was going on, 2017 was a really enjoyable year from a professional point of view. I travelled a lot for work, particularly with the Constance Hotel Group, with whom I had been contracted for two years to design a series of plant-based wellness menus. I enjoyed my work trips to a number of their luxury hotels and resorts across the Indian Ocean, meeting with their team of chefs to create delicious vegan recipes based on fresh local ingredients. I also worked with some fantastic brands and signed up for my MSc degree. However, the year was tainted by what we were going through. It was always in the background, something that we could never disconnect from. Fertility issues seem to consume you and make it difficult to plan ahead. You focus so intently on having a successful pregnancy that other aspects of life are put on hold or just fade in significance when you really want a family. All your creative and emotional energy goes into this dream and it can be exhausting. From the outside, it looked as though we were both happy, successful and getting on with our lives, but that cycle of pregnancy and devastating loss continued without reprieve. Infertility felt like a full-time job.

In June 2017, we were invited to a wedding. I'd just found out that I was pregnant following my hysteroscopy and I was feeling optimistic that it would work this time because we had apparently corrected the issue. I spent the whole night holding one full glass of wine, and if anyone said to me, 'Let's have another one,' I'd say, 'Oh, I just need to go to the bathroom, will you please hold my drink?' and when I'd come back, they'd have forgotten all about it.

I became pregnant so often that I'd frequently have to turn down invitations to events or offers of drinks. My close group of friends knew what was happening because it was an important part of our coping strategy to have trusted people to confide in. My mum and dad were amazing throughout, and Wes's cousin Jeff Ledwidge and his wife, Julie, were a huge support to us during this time. But to be honest, I found it very difficult over those few years to talk to my wider group of friends about having babies. They were all having their first and even second children, while Wes and I were still struggling, and I had such mixed emotions about it. I was so happy for my friends on their pregnancies and the safe arrival of their babies, but at the same time, I felt the most awful pang of sadness that it hadn't happened for us. It wasn't that I was jealous; I just felt despairing and lonely. And it was hard not to blame myself. I'd think, *Surely it's the most natural thing in the world. That's what our bodies as women are designed to do.* I kept coming back to the idea that my body was damaged and dysfunctional.

By mid-2017, I had contacted our fourth fertility specialist. This doctor had a particular interest in the area of reproductive immunology. As you can imagine, conducting quality randomised controlled trials into miscarriage is difficult both logistically and ethically, and there are still many unknown factors surrounding it. I was warned that the immune system in pregnancy requires more research, but despite that, I decided to take a leap of faith. After my consultation, I was advised to take a number of tests, including the Chicago blood test, which costs in excess of €1,000. This is a detailed blood immunology panel to analyse natural killer (NK) cells and Th1/Th2 (T helper cells) cytokine ratios and it's sent off to Chicago for analysis, hence the name. The human immune system is extraordinarily complex and it has been argued that the uterine immune environment is different to that of the systemic immune system as shown in a blood sample. To summarise as simply as possible, NK cells are essential for immune system defences, but in women experiencing infertility or recurrent miscarriage they've been found to be present in an increased quantity. It has been suggested that a balanced level of NK cells may support successful conception but too great an amount may indicate an imbalance in the immune system. Th1 and Th2 are considered the two major divisions of the immune system, with Th1 cytokines responding aggressively to foreign bodies or invaders deemed to be non-self and Th2 contributing to allergic reactions and responses against pathogens and parasites that do not infect cells directly. It's thought to be beneficial in pregnancy for the balance to be tipped towards a greater quantity of Th2 cytokines.

I was in the hairdresser's, hair full of foil, having my colour done, when I got the phone call with my results. The doctor said, 'Well, they were all normal except for a significant imbalance between your Th1 and Th2 cytokines.' By this stage I was more than familiar with medical jargon and I knew that cytokines are hormonal messengers responsible for biological effects in the immune system. My doctor's theory was that this imbalance was propelling my immune system into a chronically alert state, driving a fight response to attack a foreign invader, such as my husband's DNA. In a normal pregnancy, your immune response adapts to accommodate this foreign body, but my immune system wasn't doing this, it seemed. Instead, it was destroying the implanted embryo before it had a chance to develop. This made perfect sense to me and I almost collapsed into tears of relief. 'Thank you,' I repeated into the phone. 'Thank you for this answer that I've been looking for throughout the past year and a half.'

After all that we'd been through, it seemed that Wes and I finally had our answer, and I could banish all of those feelings of guilt and self-blame. There was nothing wrong with the way my reproductive system was functioning; the issue was a suspected imbalance in my immune system, which helped to make us feel a bit more hopeful. It marked a turning point in our journey, and even though we still had a long way to go, we could focus once again in a refreshed way, free of the baggage of guilt that had weighed us both down for the past couple of years. It was time to move on to a new phase.

CHAPTER 3

THE APPLIANCE OF SCIENCE

I remember being at a family party in 2016, very soon after I'd had that first miscarriage, and I was still feeling quite shocked and vulnerable. An older guest and I were chatting; we'd been discussing our families when she said, 'Surely you should be thinking about having a baby soon. What age are you?'

I was totally taken aback. 'I'm only in my early thirties,' I said, my mind busy trying to come up with a plausible explanation. 'I'm not quite ready to have a family yet – I have some more career goals to achieve.'

'Time is ticking,' she replied matter-of-factly. 'I had my first baby at twenty-two.'

I was smiling and talking casually on the outside but feeling utterly heartbroken on the inside. I'm sure the guest thought this was just harmless small talk and she could have had no idea what was going on in my world, but people often venture an opinion about other people's reproductive plans. It's such a personal subject and you never really know what's going on in another person's life, so my advice is to avoid the baby question unless the information is offered. The contents of your womb is absolutely nobody's business.

Later on, I became much more assertive about answering such questions on my terms, because I'd accepted the idea that my body wasn't capable of carrying a baby to term and that's just who I was. If I was asked about when I was thinking of having a baby, I would simply say, 'Actually, I can't physically have my own baby.' I had to do a lot of work on myself to make peace with being told that I would probably never carry my own baby, and gradually I reached the conclusion that I could still live a full and happy life without children of my own. I spent a lot of time thinking about my life and the person I am, considering what would make me feel happy and fulfilled if children didn't feature. As an animal lover, I felt that having a home full of pets would be a part of my future, and I even toyed with the idea of establishing an animal sanctuary. Living a life of purpose and making a positive impact on the lives of others in the process was my goal.

All of this was true – and it also stopped many an intrusive conversation. However, it never occurred to me until much later in our fertility journey that part of my issue might be that I didn't know how to relax. I'm sure that many women have heard this and rolled their eyes at the suggestion, but I've found it to be true. Indeed, the idea that stress may negatively impact fertility is often spoken about anecdotally. Until the first lockdown of 2020, I always felt that I had to be doing something productive. I packed my days with work, travel, workouts, study, research, meetings and emails. I pushed myself hard until I was exhausted and always needed to feel that I had achieved something with my time. I thrived on adrenaline and stress. I was a nightmare to sit down in front of a movie with because I'd either be replying to emails or snuggled into a corner of the sofa, fast asleep. It wasn't uncommon for me to make two or even three overnight trips a week to Germany for work events, all of which involved catching 7 a.m. flights. There was no middle ground. In fact, family and friends would often say it to me. 'Rosie, if you could only relax more, things might feel less overwhelming.' I didn't particularly want to hear this but, as I later discovered, relaxing really does help. The more you think about your struggles, the more you feel that there is no way out of them. It can be a vicious cycle.

In my case, there was a sense of trying to escape the reality of our situation. I was scared to relax too much and face the difficult emotions resulting from what we were going through. Perhaps I was afraid to be left alone with my own thoughts. Having nothing to do would make me do exactly that, so I would escape into work. It was a protective mechanism, I suppose. I'm still a bit guilty of it – ironically, having Sophia really helped because I had to adapt to her pace of life. And a young baby's pace is slow. A whole day could disappear just feeding her, soothing her, rocking her to sleep, going for leisurely park walks or letting her play with my jewellery, which fascinates her.

Back in 2017, I couldn't quite relax, but I was excited to begin a new medical approach. I'd been prescribed 20mg per day of Prednisolone, which is a corticosteroid. The idea was that it would suppress my immune system enough to support successful embryo implantation and development. In addition, I was advised to take a course of Humira injections, which is a tumour necrosis factor (TNF) blocker medicine designed to reduce the inflammation associated with auto-immune conditions, including Crohn's disease or rheumatoid arthritis. TNF is an inflammatory cytokine or small protein utilised by the immune system for cell signalling. Humira binds to inflammation-causing protein TNF Alpha and prevents it from engaging with other cells. My consultant had prescribed two injections over a matter of weeks, then the plan was to do a second round of Chicago tests called the 'half-Chicago' to examine specific responses of my immune system. In addition to the Humira and the steroids, I took fish oil capsules, to benefit from their anti-inflammatory EPA and DHA essential fatty acids, and a nurse came to our house regularly to administer an intralipid infusion. This was done via intravenous drip into my arm and is designed for the management of recurrent implantation failure. It's based on a fat emulsion of soybean, egg yolk phospholipids, glycerine and water. I used to sit in front of the TV for a couple of hours while it dripped into my bloodstream, as if it were a perfectly normal weeknight activity. I also had weekly acupuncture sessions designed to support fertility, and I really believed that we were doing all we could to give ourselves the best possible chance of success. I spent hours online researching various fertility treatments, poring over academic papers and reading success stories from other women on fertility forums, feeling bolstered by their positive experiences.

It's pretty hard to relax while taking a corticosteroid and I could certainly feel its effects in my body. It was like a huge surge of adrenaline, as if I'd drunk ten coffees at once, and if I were to have any chance of sleeping at night, I had to take it before seven o'clock in the morning. I avoided sugar and alcohol, which can exacerbate the bloating side effects, but after a month or two I began to notice that I was developing a puffy face and midsection, as well as mouth ulcers and headaches, apparently from the Humira injections. Still, I kept on working. I was looking at my diary recently and underneath entries like 'photo shoot' or 'travel to Germany' would be notes like 'start progesterone', 'start heparin' or 'Ovulation Day'. I really slotted our fertility journey into my everyday life, as so many of us do, I suppose, but in my case it was a coping mechanism. I felt that if I adapted to it, somehow the whole process would become normal, but in retrospect it was far from that.

Towards late 2017, I was also prescribed progesterone in a different form. I had been using pessaries, and while they weren't particularly pleasant, the injections were even less so. I had to insert a long needle directly into my glute muscle every day, which was extremely painful. I was injecting heparin into my stomach daily for blood thinning using a fine needle, but this was a *big* needle. The funny thing is, you become used to it. I was horribly bruised and sore on my tummy and bum from the injections, yet I was prepared to do whatever I could in the hope that something would eventually work. That was the mindset I had at the time, because I was so determined to have a baby. I visualised being a mum someday and dreamed of my baby's little face smiling up at me. As difficult as it was over those few years, we always had a glimmer of hope that something would work.

Wes and I developed a strong belief that we would eventually succeed, but it was massively challenging, and there were times when I'd hit a low point and feel that I was holding him back and other times where we felt much more positive. We were still young and there seemed to be nothing wrong with our fertility from the perspective of our egg and sperm quality, so we never lost hope, even though it was severely tested. I used to call our spare room 'the nursery' in the hope that one day our daughter or son would sleep there. In the meantime, we supported each other and were mutually compassionate – but, looking back, Wes did bear a lot of the emotional burden. When I'd been pregnant for a few weeks and the bleeding would start, I'd fall apart and he'd have to pick me up, hug me and put me back together. There was a lot of pressure on him to stay strong for both of us. I've noticed that when couples are going through a difficult fertility journey, more of the compassion and attention is directed towards the woman while the man is expected to be strong and cope. But Wes was losing his hopes and dreams too. I was painfully aware of that and could see that he needed reassurance and comfort.

We couldn't have got through it without our support network of close friends and family. This is such a crucial point to emphasise to any couple: it's vitally important not to suffer through it alone. When you're in the midst of the struggle, it's so difficult and intense and it feels like everything depends on your successful pregnancy. Yet you need people to say, 'Look, this is not all you are as a couple or as individuals. If it doesn't happen you still have us, you still have each other and plenty of interests and potential for a good life.' I know it's hard to think beyond parenthood when you have fertility issues and when it seems that having a baby is the only outcome that really matters, but this is when a different perspective can really help. It's not the same as glib remarks like, 'Oh, well, there's more to life than having a baby.' It's offering reassurance that, even if that much-longed-for baby doesn't arrive, you can still have a good life.

Having said all of that, I'm a perfectionist – I want everything to be just right – and this has been both a positive and a negative. I've been able to really focus on the process of asking questions and conducting my own research, but it has also contributed to our issues in a way because of my anxiety and inability to just take it easy. With conceiving and carrying our twin boys, what appears to have helped me was slowing down and relaxing.

There has been a huge change in the last few years in the conversation about fertility. Since I spoke to that wedding guest, people have realised that it's important to be sensitive. Nobody really knows what's going on in other people's private lives. Also, the discourse around fertility has changed and evolved and the conversation is now so much more open. When I went on the *Late Late Show* and spoke about our baby journey, I was overwhelmed by the love and support. Of course, there's always the odd unkind remark, but among the outpourings of positivity, they were easy to ignore. I believe that the more we can support people going through fertility issues, the better. It's all about normalising it, talking through it and accepting that infertility and miscarriage affect a huge number of us.

I understand that it's easy for me to say this now that I have my longed-for babies. I found it very difficult to talk about the problem as it was happening. No matter how open I might be, I still kept it to myself because I didn't feel I could talk about it without that happy ending. It's such a raw, sensitive topic, and I also felt a responsibility to others. I didn't want to drag them through the rollercoaster of our repeated losses and force them to emotionally invest in our struggles. For that reason, very few people knew. It was only after we had Sophia that I felt I could discuss it, because there were so many questions about surrogacy and why we chose to go down that route. I knew that I couldn't just appear one day with a baby, having not been pregnant, and say nothing. Both Wes and I felt that it was important to be honest about it.

In the aftermath of our surrogacy announcement, we heard a huge number of stories from other people. It really raised my awareness about what so many women and couples had gone through: endless rounds of IVF, stillbirths, miscarriages. People had had any number of issues, but what tied their journeys together was the range of emotions they felt, which were just like ours. There was loneliness, isolation, total devastation, a feeling of not being able to talk to anyone, that it was taboo, that it would upset others to talk about it openly or that it was too sensitive an issue for others to be able to discuss. I found that I was censoring myself in a way.

I would always tell people close to me when I was pregnant, because I wanted them to know if it didn't work, but I completely understand that many people feel they don't want to 'jinx' things until they reach the twelve-week mark. For example, I didn't announce my pregnancy with our twins until we were halfway through it because I was too nervous and grappling with a range of emotions. But I can't help feeling that this contributes to the taboo of silence around infertility or miscarriage. As a woman, perhaps you don't want the world to know about your internal functioning, but at the same time, we can't expect to have other people's support if they don't know what's happening. Now, I wish I'd been a bit more vocal. At the time we didn't talk about it to anyone outside our tight circle and we protected our privacy, but since I've been more open, there's been nothing but love and support and a sense of being on a shared journey – after all, we're just humans trying to navigate our way through life and no outcome is certain.

Back in 2017, taking my prescribed course of medication, I became pregnant in June but lost it again at six and a half weeks. I was pregnant again in August, but it didn't work out; then I got pregnant again in November and that ended in another early miscarriage. It seemed that my confidence earlier in the year that I'd managed to find the root of the problem was fading. I'd done the half-Chicago blood tests, but the results weren't conclusive, and it seemed that I was no closer to finding out what lay behind the unbreakable cycle of pregnancy and early miscarriage. Finally, early in 2018, my doctor admitted, 'Look, there's nothing much I can do for you any more. The likelihood of you ever carrying your own baby is unfortunately very low.' When a fertility expert says that to you, it's completely devastating. There's such a finality to it. You feel that you've really reached the end of the road, that you won't have your happy ending after all. I think this was the first time that I began to accept the idea that it wasn't going to happen for Wes and me.

Then, in early 2018, I contacted another consultant in London. My fifth! A friend had recommended him to me, and on our Skype call, he sounded very reassuring. 'Look,' he said to me confidently, 'I've seen this problem so many times before, don't worry, we'll get you your baby.' I was ecstatic. After all the worry and stress, here was a doctor who was breezily self-assured that he could treat me and that it would all work out. In hindsight, I probably ought to have been more cautious. After all, if four other doctors had been baffled by my case, why was this one so sure he could fix it? I have since learned that some fertility clinics can be over-optimistic; after all, who wants to tell an anxious woman or couple that they haven't got a chance? Nobody really wants to be in a position of dashing hopes, do they? But back then, I was desperate.

'Please send over all of your medical reports and test results – anything that's of any use to me – via email,' he instructed. Based on those, he would organise a new round of blood tests and he would analyse the results. I rang his secretary a few days later and left a voicemail, eager to find out what his feedback would be, but received no response. I rang and emailed a few times more, but still heard nothing. That doctor never got back to me. Now, I think that he saw my test results and felt that, actually, I wasn't treatable after all, but at the time it was a huge letdown. Our hopes had been raised so high only to be crushed again. This is a sadly common story among couples who have had fertility issues, and the only thing I can really say is I know how you feel. It can and does happen, and the only thing to do is reach out to others for support and do as much research as you can on doctors and clinics.

I felt very down after that. I'd covered every angle with every consultant I'd seen, I'd completed as much reading about infertility as I could, I'd taken all the medication I'd been prescribed and I still had no baby. I thought back to the conversation that I'd had with Wes months before, where I'd urged him to leave me and he'd said, 'We can still have a good life, Rosie.' Maybe I would have to accept that now. I would have to learn to live my life without a baby, without a family. It would take time to adjust to it, but somehow, we'd manage.

But before I put the previous two years of struggle behind me, I decided to have a chat with one of the original doctors I'd seen. Even though he hadn't been able to help, I'd really liked him and thought that at least he would be honest with me. In February 2018, I sat in his office and said, 'We've seen everyone and tried everything and we're at a point now where we don't know what we can do – we've run out of options.'

He sat back in his chair and thought for a bit before saying, 'I'd agree that I can't see what more could be done for you.' I knew that IVF was not an option because I could become pregnant without problems, but something was happening to prevent the embryo from developing normally and no doctor had been able to get to the bottom of it.

'What do you think about surrogacy?' I said. I had been thinking about the possibility for a while, but asking another woman to carry and give birth your child is a huge decision to make and I hadn't felt ready to accept that. Now, though, I felt that I might be.

'Well,' he replied, 'it's a feasible option for a couple like you who have time on your side. It's not an egg quantity or quality issue from what I can see, so that might well be a solution.' We both agreed that I'd give it some thought, and I left feeling a tiny bit more hopeful. Surrogacy is complicated, both legally and psychologically, and the idea of a stranger in a different country walking around pregnant with my baby honestly horrified me, but after everything we'd been through, it seemed like our only hope of having a family.

The irony is, I got pregnant again that month during a family holiday. I thought, wouldn't it be funny if this worked out, just as we'd given up? Sadly, it didn't. So, Wes and I picked ourselves up, dusted ourselves off and said, 'We're going to look at surrogacy.' We took a few weeks to really think hard about it and do some research. I had to make what felt like the most difficult decision of my life so far: would I be able to cope with seeing another woman pregnant with the child that I so desperately wanted to carry? I wasn't sure that I would be strong enough for everything that surrogacy entailed, but ultimately it had become our only option, and in March 2018, we decided that we were ready.

Are you thinking of having a family?' Nobody ever asked Wes, 'I hope work is going well, but when are you going to take time off to have a family?' There is a double standard here, something I'm sure other couples experience.

Those types of judgement do affect you. After a while I began to think, Do people assume I'm really selfish, swanning around the Indian Ocean, putting glossy photos up on social media? Do they think that I'm simply putting my career first? Even though I knew that the only people who mattered in this story were Wes and me (and our families, of course) I'd have to come up with answers as to why I wasn't settling down and starting a family.

Another difficult aspect of infertility that took me by surprise at the time was seeing photos of happy family occasions on Facebook or Instagram. Whether it was Christmas, Easter, Mother's or Father's Day, social media would be flooded with beautiful pictures of babies and toddlers with their proud parents and I found this heartbreaking to see. It seemed so unfair that we were desperately trying everything to have a baby while it seemed to happen easily for others. I realise now from speaking about our experiences that far more couples have faced fertility issues than I ever realised. But it also underlined for me that society is very much centred around families and children. It seems that when you don't have a baby, family-friendly facilities and activities are everywhere. Of course, that's wonderful, but it can be so isolating for those who don't have children. I'm very conscious now, especially when posting about Sophia online, that there are so many people who would love to become a mum or dad. I feel that experiencing both aspects has made me much more empathic and compassionate towards others because we all have our struggles in some form or other.

In retrospect, I realise that just over two years on a fertility journey might not seem like an awfully long time, but when you're in the midst of it, living according to your monthly cycle and watching your friends have children, the time feels like an eternity. Mum tried to put things in perspective for me, giving me a big hug and saying, 'You know, you've had so much go your way in your life that when something doesn't happen for you it can be difficult, but you have to keep up the hope and the faith that it will.' She was right, of course. I've always been the kind of person who thought that if I put in the hard work and intelligent effort and focused on what I had to do to achieve something, whether it was a career goal, an academic goal or a relationship goal, I'd get there. That's what makes infertility so difficult to accept and understand.

However, when Wes and I talked about the issue of surrogacy, we both knew that it had to be a joint commitment. Even though I had taken the lead so far in terms of researching our options, we wanted to approach this new phase as a couple. I had been through a difficult period of feeling that I was in some way defective, preventing Wes from having a family, but I'd worked hard to combat the self-blame. We knew how critically important it would be to fully support each other and work as a team, which is vital for any couple going through fertility issues.

At this stage, Wes and I didn't know where to even begin when it came to gestational surrogacy, which involves another woman carrying and delivering a child for an individual or a couple. It felt incredibly overwhelming, and although we had heard about other couples going through the process, we knew very little about how it worked. This was probably a positive thing, in hindsight, because it's a lengthy, complex, difficult process, despite how positive an experience it ultimately was for us. We feel so lucky that our story had a happy ending and that surrogacy is a feasible route to parenthood thanks to the wonders of modern medical science and the women who agree to carry another couple's baby, but it's by no means the easy option financially, emotionally or practically.

Following some research, we decided that the most important first step would be to establish our legal rights, so we made an appointment with a solicitor who specialises in surrogacy law. We drove into Dublin city centre on a freezing cold day in March 2018; little snowflakes were falling as we walked briskly towards the office block. It was the week of the Beast from the East, and although the real snow had yet to arrive, the streets were deserted. It felt as if the whole world was holding its breath, just like we were.

The solicitor was extremely helpful, providing us with an overview of the process from a legal perspective, outlining which countries have surrogacy programmes and what they entail. Those of you who have experienced the process will know that a limited number of countries permit surrogacy. Some will only allow 'altruistic' surrogacy, where no money apart from medical and living expenses changes hands; others permit commercial surrogacy. Some countries, such as Ukraine, will only allow heterosexual couples on their programmes, so many gay couples go to Canada or the United States. She suggested Ukraine, as we were a married heterosexual couple, and she'd had clients who'd had great success there.

The solicitor talked us through the checklist of what would be needed for the Ukrainian programme and showed us a list of clinics and agencies. In Ukraine, an agency will run the legal side of the programme, select the surrogate and act as the coordinator between the parents and surrogate. The agency will partner with a fertility clinic, who will run the medical side of it, including the egg retrieval, embryo transfer and scans.

We had a great deal to think about and it certainly didn't appear to be the easy route to parenthood. The solicitor had made it clear to us that surrogacy would cost a lot of money. The way we looked at it was that it was saveable for, in the same way you might save for a wedding or a car or a mortgage. Everyone has different priorities in life and they'll save for what they consider valuable. We were prepared and willing to pay as much as it took for this hugely important next step in our lives. We decided on Ukraine because their requirements were very clear and we felt comfortable with the legal and medical framework. We would know what paperwork we'd have to supply and what would be required both from us and from the surrogate. We also made the decision to opt for commercial gestational surrogacy, where a fee would be paid to the agency – and ultimately to the surrogate. We felt that viewing it as more of a 'business arrangement' might help to reduce or dilute the emotional load for us and the surrogate. Perhaps this seems a bit clinical, but we didn't take the decision lightly. We knew that we were asking another woman, a stranger at that, to carry our biological child. There would be emotions on both sides – how could there not be? But we felt that the system in Ukraine ensured that everyone would understand their rights and be treated fairly.

The next step was to find an agency. Here, there was no special magic involved, just Google. I spent a lot of time looking through discussion threads and message boards about various agencies in Ukraine, marvelling that people were talking about their experiences with such honesty. I selected a few agencies, then emailed them, explaining our situation. I was drawn to one agency in particular because I was impressed by their response and by the detailed PDF they provided. It was twelve pages in total, outlining exactly what would be required and the specific process involved for different types of surrogacy – for example, whether or not couples planned to use donor eggs or sperm, or their own biological material as Wes and I did.

The first step required by the agency was proof of our identities and marital status. We obtained a copy of our original marriage certificate to have notarised and stamped with the required 'Apostille' stamp, which is a certificate issued by the Department of Foreign Affairs and Trade to verify the authenticity of a document. I went into a little office on the quays close to Dublin's O'Connell Street for the official stamp, before scanning the certificate and emailing it to the agency. We had to do the same with our birth certificates and passports.

Next, we moved our focus onto the extensive list of medical requirements. Wes and I needed to medically prove that we were free from infectious diseases and sexually transmitted diseases and show that we were genetically normal via karyotype testing, which can diagnose chromosomal abnormalities. I was asked to book an appointment with a consultant in genetic haematology because of my inherited blood-clotting condition and have blood tests done by him, the results of which took some time. I redid my smear test and on one particular day I was advised to drive to the virology lab in UCD with a blood sample because it was quicker than waiting for a courier to collect it. Another test for a type of bacterial infection had to be sent to a lab in Greece. Wes had a complete sperm analysis, a chest X-ray to establish the absence of tuberculosis and his blood group and rhesus factor tested. I had a wide range of blood coagulation and hormone tests, in addition to a breast ultrasound and ovarian scan to establish that I didn't have cysts and was healthy enough to undergo the hormone injections required by the egg-retrieval process. My GP also had to confirm by letter that she knew of no medical reason for me not to be accepted onto the surrogacy programme. Ultimately, we both had to prove that our biological material was healthy, so that transferral into the surrogate wouldn't cause her to develop any health issues. It was an intimidatingly long list and it took Wes and me six months to complete with repeat visits to our doctors and various specialists, but we felt reassured by the level of detail. The agency was taking every step to ensure that the health and well-being of both parties would be protected.

We had had some of the tests done before applying for surrogacy, but the clinic in Kiev specified that they had to be recent, within the last three or six months depending on the test. It was quite a logistical challenge because the term of validity of some of the tests had expired by the time we got the results of others, so they needed to be repeated. Sometimes I felt as though I was on an obstacle course, having just cleared one big jump before having to climb another. Thankfully, I have a wonderfully supportive and understanding GP, who helped me by undertaking as many of the tests as she could and advising where I could have the other tests done. At one point, I was seeing her up to three times a week either for a blood test or to collect results, which all had to be signed and stamped by the relevant clinic. It was intense, to say the least.

The extent of the tests required from us really highlighted the dramatic difference between the natural process of pregnancy and this incredibly scientific experience. As humans, we think we can do anything, but so much of life is outside our control.

The irony was that I actually became pregnant in spring 2018, as we were beginning our surrogacy journey. Despite presuming that it would follow the usual pattern and fail to develop, I couldn't help wishing that it would so we could leave the complex world of surrogacy behind us. Even at that early stage, the process seemed endless and the outcome so uncertain. I remembered a conversation that I'd had with a nurse in 2017. She'd come to the house to administer the intralipid infusion, and I told her that if I couldn't carry my own baby I'd been thinking about surrogacy as a possible option. 'Really?' she said. 'Surrogacy is extreme, though, isn't it?' Now, I thought, maybe it *is* extreme. All of the tests, the contracts, the verifications, the fact that I would be entrusting this baby to another woman. What if there was one more chance? I thought. What if this pregnancy did work? I didn't want to hope for too much, to invest in it only to be disappointed once more, so when it lasted six-and-a-half weeks I was philosophical. We'd just have to pick ourselves up again and keep going.

Finally, by the autumn of 2018 the tests were complete and we were ready to move to the next stage of the process, the signing of the contracts. In October, we were sent all of the contracts we'd need to read over, eleven or twelve in total, in both English and Ukrainian. We sought the help of a solicitor, as each page of the extensive contracts had to be signed individually and returned via email. However, it was reassuring to have this legal framework established and documents to protect the rights of each party involved.

Among all of this, I had applied for a full-time Master of Science degree in Personalised Nutrition online through Middlesex University, but there was a method to my madness. I wanted to distract myself from the whole process and from focusing too intently on something that might not work out. I also felt that I badly needed time out to hide away from the world and concentrate on my studies and work obligations. I realise now that part of me was trying to avoid seeing people and having to answer potentially upsetting and awkward questions about baby plans. I also felt that I had put my life on hold to a certain extent in 2017 and wanted to make the most of my year. Looking back, I wonder how I coped with the pressure of it all, but it was a welcome distraction from the emotional intensity of the process. We had such a challenging time ahead of us that I could only focus on the next step, celebrating each small victory along the way.

On 11 November 2018, we finally signed and scanned the contracts and emailed them to the agency, then received that precious and long-awaited email accepting us onto the surrogacy programme. This was after the best part of a year of blood tests, scans, paperwork and almost daily emails with various members of the team in Ukraine. The next day, I sent over the entire file of physical documents, including our stamped blood test results, the contracts and various certificates, via registered post. I couldn't rest for the next two weeks while waiting for the email to confirm its arrival in Kiev and was immensely relieved when I was told that the package had safely reached its destination. If it had got lost on the way there, we'd have been back to square one. I couldn't even bear to think about going through the whole process again. My maternal grandmother, Marion Morley (née Nairn), had passed away on 11 November 2005, and it gave me comfort and encouragement to think that perhaps she was, in some way, a part of that special day and with us on our journey.

I would love to say that after all of this we had a relaxing Christmas, but I was in the stressed-out depths of writing my master's dissertation, which was due in mid-January, and Wes had just opened his new business, the Carlton Casino Club, in November, so he was kept extremely busy with that. I can still remember researching my dissertation among all of the uncertainty with contracts and forms and asking Wes to sign them when he came home after long days at the office. At the time, you somehow get used to it and feel that it's normal to be anxious and stressed all the time, but now I look back and think, how did we get through that?

My dissertation was due to be submitted on 15 January 2019, and the week before, I received another email from the agency. They had begun the search for a surrogate and were to interview a woman the following week. It all suddenly began to feel very real. The agency has a database of possible candidates from all over Ukraine, and women interested in potentially becoming surrogates can apply. However, they have strict criteria for selecting prospective surrogates. They're required to be within a certain age range. They must already have a healthy child born through a normal vaginal delivery after an uncomplicated pregnancy. They need to have no medical history of adverse issues in pregnancy, a clean bill of health and be non-smokers and non-drinkers.

By sheer serendipity, I handed in my dissertation on the same day that we heard about our potential surrogate – a memorable day for Wes and me. I submitted it at midday, flew off to Mauritius on a working holiday with the Constance Hotel Group at 1.30 that afternoon and, just before our plane took off, my phone pinged with the email from the agency confirming that they were very happy to recommend this woman to us. I scanned the form showing me her details and photographs, hands shaking with a heady mix of excitement and fear of the unknown. This might be the woman who grows and gives birth to our child.

It felt strange to look at those stark details and imagine the woman who lay behind them. We were told that she seemed very nice and responsible, had a two-year-old of her own, and a few other basic details including her age and profession, but nothing more than that. Some parents will form a closer bond with their surrogate, exchanging photos and little bits of news, and while we were offered the opportunity to meet her, we decided not to. We didn't want to upset her by being overbearing or by crossing any boundaries, but also, we wanted to protect ourselves a little bit. We were both used to disappointment and couldn't fully trust in the process just yet. I was also a little scared about discovering more about her on a human level, and it felt somehow safer to view our relationship with her as a business one. I've found that it's essential to protect your emotional well-being and mental health, particularly when faced with a potentially life-changing event.

For me, the only way forward was never to fully believe that our family dream would come true, that there would be a happy outcome to this gruelling process. It might seem illogical, but it was my way of protecting myself – to take things step by step, to celebrate each small victory along the way, but never to look too far ahead. I compartmentalised it, telling myself, 'The next step we have to take is this … and the next one is this …' never looking any further into the future. It's such a long process and demands so much of your emotional energy and resilience as a person and as a couple that the best way through it seems to be to take it in baby steps. And so, we did. The next step in our surrogacy journey would take us to Kiev for the all-important egg-retrieval process. We were well and truly on our way.

CHAPTER 5

PINK SPRINKLES

Winter in Kiev is dark and very cold. The temperature tends to hover in the minus figures and it snows quite a lot, but none of this bothered me as I made my final preparations to travel there for the egg-retrieval part of the surrogacy process. I had been told that I'd need to spend around two weeks in the city for the entire procedure so I was well prepared, with my snow boots, guidebooks and winter clothing, not to mention the company of Mum, who was coming to support me for the first week before Wes would fly out.

I'd actually been to the city before, back in 2011, when I'd been on the judging panel of Miss Ukraine, along with

Paris Hilton and 'The Muscles from Brussels', Jean-Claude Van Damme. Van Damme was charming and funny and Paris was very sweet and chatty. It was a relaxed, fun work trip and very different to this, my second visit.

I'd begun to prepare for the egg-retrieval process a couple of weeks before with a scan of my ovaries to ensure that they looked healthy and there were no cysts or other complications. The clinic had told me that the egg-retrieval cycle must be tied into my own menstrual cycle, so I would go to Kiev in early February. Before that, they asked me to take the contraceptive pill for three to four weeks to help regulate my cycle and presumably avoid any chance of pregnancy. My GP has always discouraged me from taking the pill because of my family history of blood clots, so I returned to the consultant haematologist for a letter permitting me to take it, with the recommendation that I also take daily aspirin and self-injected heparin to guard against clotting.

On Monday 4 February 2019, Mum and I flew via Frankfurt to Kiev. We'd told very few people the real reason I was going; I hadn't even told my granny, which made me feel guilty because we're very close. Mum had to make up an excuse that we were going on a work-related trip for Wes's new business, and we felt uncomfortable with the dishonesty, but I knew that it was for the best. Looking back, I think it was a form of self-protection. I didn't want to raise people's hopes or for them to invest in the outcome of this journey only for it not to work. Judgements didn't bother me at that stage because I'd become very confident about saying that I wasn't able to have my own baby, but the last thing I wanted was to disappoint those closest to me.

The science nerd in me found the whole process very interesting even if, as a woman, it all felt pretty invasive. When you undertake something like surrogacy or IVF, your body is viewed from a medical perspective, and you quickly learn that feeling shy is a waste of time and energy. I thought about how much detail to include when I was writing this, but decided in the end that I'd leave nothing out. I really want to describe the process I went through as best I can and to represent what's involved for women having a baby with the necessary assistance of medical science.

I was asked to stop taking the contraceptive pill a day or two after I'd arrived so that my period would appear on schedule. Of course, it didn't! To help things along, I was given an injection of progesterone by the clinic to stimulate my period, and they felt confident that it would work. While we were waiting, Mum and I spent a week getting to know Kiev together. It was such a nice mother–daughter bonding experience and I have wonderful memories of our time there. The city looked beautiful in the snow and we explored the fabulously decorative cathedrals, wandered around museums and ate delicious meals. The food scene in Kiev is excellent, and I was delighted at the number of restaurants that cater for vegans and vegetarians. We even watched the Irish rugby team beat Scotland 22-13 on 9 February while we sat in an

Irish pub. Obviously, though, the main reason we were there was to get on with the egg-retrieval process and my period still wasn't coming. I was in constant touch with the clinic and they kept saying, 'Give it a few more days. We can't start the egg-ripening process until it begins.' The irony is that it probably wasn't appearing because of my anxiety about it appearing. It just goes to show that we're often at the mercy of our own bodies and we can't control them in the way that we'd like.

After a week of sightseeing and waiting, it was time for Mum to fly home. Thankfully, Wes was joining me for the second week, but even so, I remember feeling tearful when saying goodbye to Mum because we'd had such a lovely girly week together and she'd been so supportive. I waved her off in the hotel lobby and had three hours to wait until Wes's flight arrived. And what do you know? My period arrived in that three-hour window. When my mother heard later that day, she laughed and said, 'That's so typical! All it took was for me to leave and Wes to arrive for it all to start happening.' There's probably some truth to that; perhaps subconsciously I'd been waiting for Wes, my other half in this journey, before I felt ready.

In a state of relief and excitement, I contacted the clinic and they said, 'Great. Come in tomorrow morning and we'll get started.' By 'get started' they meant on the process of maturing and harvesting my eggs. It was a strange feeling to actually begin, because it's something we had thought about for so long. As a woman, you've prepared medically, mentally, emotionally and, now, physically – yet there's no guarantee that it will work. It's not like most other contracts in life, which tend to guarantee an end result. We were interrupting nature with science – a dichotomy that has to work in tandem for this process to succeed.

We began on 13 February with my first 200ml injection of GONAL-f administered at the clinic to start the process of stimulating my ovaries to mature eggs in a larger quantity than my body normally would each month. The doctor offered to inject for me, but I was so used to my daily heparin injections that I was quite happy to do it myself. The next day, I administered another 200ml injection of GONAL-f, and throughout the entire process I was observed carefully for any symptoms of ovarian hyperstimulation syndrome, which is an exaggerated reaction by the ovaries to excess hormones, causing swelling and pain. It can be very dangerous, even life-threatening. I had a scan of my ovaries every second day to make sure no issues were arising and to check the growth of my follicles. The process was incredibly invasive. All the scans involve a transvaginal probe, which isn't particularly pleasant, but the clinic staff were great. It was run more or less totally by women and I felt comfortable and also reassured by their professionalism. And, of course, Wes was very supportive and hoping as much as I was that we'd have a successful outcome.

The entire process of maturing my eggs took another ten days, time which Wes and I spent wandering around the city, enjoying the cafés, shops and museums. I was certainly getting to know the place well at that stage. Because so few people knew that we were there, we had the feeling that we were hidden away from the world, and we needed that sense of anonymity, I think, that quietness, while we waited for things to happen. However, in the final four days of the egg-stimulation process, my ovaries were so swollen that I found it quite uncomfortable to walk around. I felt as though I were carrying bags of marbles in my abdomen. Looking back, though, I'm grateful for those few days because it was as if I was carrying Sophia in my body in a very palpable way. It is comforting to think that she was a part of me, that she had been in my body my whole life as a little egg – and in my mother's body too, as I was developing *in utero*. I find that aspect of maternal lineage absolutely incredible. This also helped to ameliorate some of the guilt I felt about not being capable of carrying her and giving birth to her and made me feel a part of the whole process.

On 20 February, the clinic confirmed that my eggs were ready to be harvested. However, unlike in nature, this had to follow a strict schedule to prevent ovulation happening before the procedure to extract my eggs. The danger when you get to this point is that your body will ovulate and everything will be lost. This ended up being quite funny as I stood in the hotel bathroom, two syringes full of Cetrotide (which blocks the egg-releasing hormone) on the edge of the sink. I was to take them at 11.30 p.m. exactly, not a moment sooner or later. The medical coordinator of the clinic was messaging me on WhatsApp saying, 'OK, do it now, and let me know when you've done it!' At exactly 11.30 p.m., I cleaned the area on my tummy with the cleansing pad and injected myself twice.

The next important day on our journey was 22 February 2019, when my precious eggs were retrieved. I had been assured by the doctor that I had a healthy quantity of follicles in each ovary, which hopefully would yield mature eggs. Wes and I headed into the clinic early that morning in a state of nervous anticipation. I would be knocked out for an hour while Wes would simply have to go off with a little container and do his part, a cinch compared to mine. 'Look at you,' I joked. 'I have to go through all of this and all you have to do is pleasure yourself!' Obviously, it's all due to the way we are biologically designed, but it does show that women's bodies generally have to endure so much more medical invasion and investigation than those of men.

I changed into a hospital gown and one of the nurses brought me into the theatre where the procedure would take place. There, I was helped onto a cold, blue birthing chair, my legs placed in stirrups that lifted them high into the air. It certainly wasn't ladylike, but I tried to relax as the three nurses and the surgeon milled around me, filling in forms. At this stage, I was used to all of it. Anyone who has been through the fertility system will know that you lose any self-consciousness pretty quickly. When it comes to the human body, the medics have to do their job and embarrassment doesn't come into it.

I was given IV sedation via a needle into the back of my hand and the last thing I remember was the doctor smiling at me and speaking in Ukrainian as I drifted off. For egg-retrieval procedures, a propofol-based sedation medication is often used so that the patient falls into a deep sleep and doesn't feel a thing. The process takes twenty to thirty minutes and involves pushing a narrow needle with a catheter through the vaginal wall into the ovary and gently sucking out the eggs before storing them in a nutritive liquid, a fluid that's chemically similar to that of your own body. The procedure was successful and I woke up half an hour later in the recovery room, Wes at my bedside. The first thing I said was, 'Wes, did you get your job done?'

He replied, 'Yes, Rosie, you don't need to worry about me! Worry about yourself.' We still laugh about that.

I was in a little bit of discomfort, so I was given painkillers, hooked up to a drip and told to rest for a while in bed. I must have been tired because I nodded off immediately. After a couple of hours, I felt fully revived and the anaesthetic had worn off, so we rang for a taxi back to the hotel. We relaxed in the room for a little while, feeling relieved that it was all over, but then we decided to go out to celebrate. Nothing too energetic – just dinner with a glass of champagne – yet it felt significant to both of us. We couldn't believe that the procedure was finished and that chapter of our journey was complete. Our physical contribution had concluded and the next part of the process was the responsibility of the clinic and our gestational surrogate. The clinic told us they had retrieved twenty-three eggs and they were very happy with the quantity, but the emotion both of us felt was one of sheer relief. In a series of small victories, this was a huge one for us, a real milestone.

After another couple of days and a further trip to the clinic for a check-up and a final IV drip to help eliminate the sedative from my system, we were ready to go home. We'd been in Kiev for almost three weeks at that stage, walking the length and breadth of the city, enjoying quiet time together, but never forgetting the purpose of our visit. It was another step in the right direction, another obstacle cleared to bring us closer to our goal.

February is a quiet month socially and many people are still in hibernation mode, so we slipped back home as quietly as we'd left at the beginning of the month. All we had to do now was wait to see if the process of fertilising the eggs was successful and how many would develop into blastocysts over a five-day period. Of my twenty-three eggs, twenty were fertilised, so the clinic was satisfied. The embryos would be placed in liquid nitrogen until our surrogate reached the recommended point in her hormone-regulated cycle, using supplemental progesterone to prepare her uterine lining for implantation. Then two would be thawed and transferred into her womb.

*

I was exhausted when we returned from Kiev, but I only realised just how tired I was when I picked up flu two days after we came home. I seldom get ill, but after the anxiety and stress of the previous three weeks, I was obviously very run-down. I'd put so much energy into the trip, both emotionally and physically, that as soon as I relaxed it hit me hard. I spent the next week in bed, reading, napping and watching Netflix. I didn't even have the mental energy left to worry about when the egg transferral procedure into our gestational surrogate would take place, and whether all of our hard work, time and money would be worth it.

On 4 March, the clinic informed me by email that a decent number of blastocysts had developed into embryos and had been frozen on day five. They had been graded into numbers and letters according to their quality and degree of expansion, although an embryo grade is only indicative of its potential ability to implant in the uterus. We decided to transfer the two best-quality embryos – a 2AA and a 2-3BB. We were recommended to have two transferred in case one doesn't implant – and if you're not afraid of multiple pregnancies. Wes and I would have been thrilled with a single baby, but I'd been secretly hoping for twins, believe it or not, thinking that it would be wonderful to have a ready-made family. Be careful what you wish for, eh?

The clinic planned and prepped for the transfer procedure to take place on 12 March and informed me that afternoon that it had gone well and that our surrogate was feeling positive and excited about the whole process. It felt so odd to be at home in Ireland while a stranger thousands of miles away was having our embryos transferred into her body. I felt utterly powerless and a little bit scared. We would find out on 26 March whether or not our surrogate was pregnant, and for the couple of nights before that date, I was a bundle of nerves. I couldn't sleep and lay awake all night thinking, is she, isn't she? I tried to rationalise my jumbled thoughts, to say to myself that the process can sometimes take a few attempts, and if this one didn't work, we had embryos left over and we could just try again, but I was desperate for something to work out for us just this once. I didn't want to lose faith in a process that had taken so much courage to pursue.

I was shaking when I opened the email on 26 March. I couldn't face reading it for a few seconds, peering through my fingers at the words on the screen. When I saw the sentence, 'I'm so happy to bring this wonderful news to you,' I burst into tears. Our gestational surrogate was pregnant. There was a lot of jumping up and down and hugging and more tears. It was such a big day for both of us. We'd been through enough to know that a positive pregnancy test doesn't mean a baby, but her hCG level looked good, and for the first time in the whole process, we hoped. Just a tiny bit.

However, even though the clinic had reassured us that everything was going according to plan, I couldn't shed my anxiety. I expected that at any moment somebody would ring me and say, 'She's lost the pregnancy.' After everything we'd been through, I was set up for disappointment. I couldn't even begin to believe that it would work. It's terrible to live like that, really stressful. So, I did what I always do when I feel stressed, which is to make myself even more busy. The distraction worked for both of us as we whizzed around, visiting my brothers in London, working hard, attending weddings and events, living our lives in two-week increments, waiting for the all-important six-week scan when we hoped to see a heartbeat.

I had a Pilates class on the morning of 8 April, and as I was walking out of the studio afterwards, my phone pinged with an email from the clinic. The surrogate had just had her six-week scan and they were delighted to tell me that they'd detected a tiny heartbeat. Wow! I couldn't believe it. It seemed incredible, especially as I had never reached the point of detecting a heartbeat in any of my failed pregnancies. When the clinic emailed me the scan pictures, I found it extraordinary to think that this tiny kidney bean might eventually become a little person. Our little person. It was another huge moment, another victory to add to all the others.

I know that I've spoken about the problems that come with keeping early pregnancy a secret. The culture of silence can make people who go through miscarriage feel that they are all alone, when support and compassion from others is such a crucial part of the healing process. Wes and I certainly felt this way, but this time we made a conscious choice to keep our secret. It was the only means we had of managing our own expectations, and also of not disappointing our families and friends. I felt that I couldn't drag them yet again through the whole spectrum of emotions that comes with pregnancy followed by loss. I did break this rule when I went on a hen-party trip to Majorca in April, though; I couldn't keep that secret to myself while holidaying for a weekend with people I've known for years. They were thrilled for us, of course, but apart from that, Wes and I were determined to keep our news quiet until the twelve-week point.

We were staying with Mum and Dad in Enniskerry when the eight-week pregnancy update arrived, on Easter Monday 22 April. It was a beautiful day and I'd taken breakfast outside to eat at the garden table in the sunshine when the email came through. There was Sophia's tiny shape on the scan photos, and we were reassured that she was growing normally and that our surrogate was feeling well. My brother Michael and his fiancée, Mary, were visiting from London, but somehow I managed to keep it to myself, even though I was desperate to share my excitement. The funny thing is that when we did tell them at twelve weeks, they said, 'You heard that news on Easter Monday and you didn't even tell us!' They were joking, of course, but I hadn't told them earlier because I wanted to protect them in case anything went wrong. When I'd had that first miscarriage in 2016, it had been Michael I'd rung in LA and I didn't want to put him through anything like that again. I didn't want him to have to deal with our sadness.

My Mum knew everything, of course, because she'd been with me every step of the way. In fact, I can still remember her sticking her head out the bedroom window that Easter Monday and saying, 'Well, any emails yet?' Dad knew all about what was happening too and was incredibly supportive, but I think he was anxious about getting too emotionally invested in case it all went wrong. Something like this really is a family affair and everyone feels the emotional load of it, not just the couple involved.

I approached the date of our ten-week scan with trepidation. I've had friends who've lost pregnancies at ten weeks, so it felt like a vulnerable point and I was anxious. Even though that scan result arrived as normal and everything was looking good, I remember just wishing the next two weeks away to the twelve-week mark. I was living from scan to scan, in chunks of two weeks, and elated at the beginning of the fortnight when everything was OK. I'd be on a high for the next week or so, then begin to worry as the second week came into view. I'd spend the whole of the second week trying to control my impulse to think the worst. I felt as if I were holding my breath, waiting for the next scan when I could exhale once more.

The critical twelve-week scan was due on 20 May. I was at work, doing a big press day for TanOrganic, and we'd set up in a hotel to introduce the new campaign to a selection of journalists. I could hardly concentrate but, somehow, I put on a brave face, trying to ignore any buzzing from my phone and focusing on being as present and professional as possible. The team and I had stopped for lunch and were sitting around the table chatting when an email arrived to my phone. I nearly dropped it in my excitement, saying, 'Just a moment, I have to run to the bathroom!' I raced downstairs and clicked into it, fingers slipping over the buttons as I tapped.

And there she was, as clear as day. I stared at the scan picture, eyes wide in amazement, looking at her tiny spine, her little legs and the developing bones of her jaw and face. I couldn't take it in – *There's an actual baby in there and it's our baby*, I thought. I stood there and I cried, big fat tears splashing down my cheeks. After all the waiting and hoping, it was suddenly becoming real. I let myself take it all in, then realised that I'd been gone a while so I had to pull myself together and get on with real life. I called Wes quickly and then my mum, whispering down the line, my voice shaking. I sent on the precious picture, then bolted back upstairs. I spent the rest of the afternoon doing interviews with journalists about TanOrganic, trying to appear calm and collected, but my brain was whirring away. That was my life, smiling through what was really happening in the background.

I looked at the scan pictures over and over again during the next few days, finding it extraordinary that this was the result of our trip to Kiev only a few months before. Nature is incredible in the way a human being can grow from just a collection of cells. I was fascinated by the speed of her growth, from that tiny kidney bean to a little human complete with functioning organs. I put her various scans together to see how quickly she'd grown and it really astonished me. At twelve weeks old, she was only three inches long, but she was a fully formed tiny person. Our baby.

The scan picture also brought up a lot of uncomfortable feelings for me. I wondered how something so perfect could grow in the surrogate's body and not in mine. I found myself wondering about the woman who had agreed to carry our genetic child and what she was going through. Did she feel as I had done during my pregnancies, short though they were? Was she excited, happy or worried? Of course, we could have met her had we wanted to, but something made me feel that this wasn't the best approach for either of us. I didn't want her to feel pressured in any way or to feel that she owed us anything, but deep down, I knew there was another reason; I was so desperate to carry Sophia that I found it hard to think about another woman carrying her for me. It compounded my feelings of inadequacy and the sense I had that my body was dysfunctional.

Nonetheless, it was such a relief to be able to share our secret at the twelve-week stage. Wes and I felt as though a weight had been lifted off our shoulders. We sent our scan pictures and FaceTimed my brothers in London to tell them and there were lots of tears of happiness. As the weeks wore on, the photos were replaced by 3D and 4D videos of little

Sophia bouncing around, her body growing and taking shape before our eyes.

The next big surprise came at sixteen weeks, when we found out that we were having a girl. Wes and I had no preference for either a boy or a girl – our focus was on having a healthy baby – but at the same time, it felt very special. I am the eldest in my family and Mum and I are very close. I hoped to have the same close relationship with my daughter and felt it would be like history repeating itself. We decided to mark it by having a little gender-reveal party with our families – just our parents, whom we gathered with in Enniskerry. I bought a cake and cut a hole in the middle, which I filled with pink sprinkles, then covered up with cake. Very crafty! When I cut it open to reveal the colour, everyone was thrilled. Dad broke out the champagne and we gave a toast to this wonderful piece of news. Still, even then I was careful to keep a part of myself back to guard against disappointment. We'd been so focused on the here and now for so long, afraid to think too much into the future, that even though finding out the gender of our child was definitely worth celebrating, I never felt that I could fully relax. Now, I wonder if I might have been more relaxed had I been carrying the baby myself, but even with our twin boys, I felt some anxiety for much of the pregnancy. Every pregnancy carries with it uncertainty, of course, but Wes and I had had our hopes raised so often, before being dashed again, that we were almost afraid to look too far ahead. By coincidence,

I found out that we were having a girl on 11 June 2019 and just one year later, on 8 June 2020, I'd find out that I was expecting twin boys. If you'd told me that was what my future held, I'd have said you were mad!

The twenty-week scan was due around 11 July, the same day that I graduated from Middlesex University with my MSc. We had flown to London for the ceremony, my mind, as ever, half-focused on the other huge event in my life. This scan is called the 'anomaly' or 'anatomy' scan, because it's generally at this point that any problems with the developing baby are spotted. The surrogate had had blood tests and the Nuchal Fold test, which tests for Down syndrome, a couple of months before and all had been well, but this was the big one. When we received the news that everything was looking normal, we were ecstatic. We could now have a double celebration. I felt that two big parts of my life had somehow come together in a really positive way and that maybe, just maybe, I could finally breathe.

From that point on, the scans became four-weekly and they were all very reassuring. Twenty-four weeks passed, then twenty-eight and thirty-two. Sophia was growing normally, our surrogate was in good health and all was well. As we passed the twenty-four-week mark, which is considered the first week of viability, I began to gradually relax. If the baby arrived now, I reasoned, with good medical care she would survive. This might seem a bit dramatic, but friends of mine who have had 'normal' pregnancies have told me they felt the same. It's a landmark for parents-to-be, a point where hopes and dreams can begin to take some kind of shape. All the same, I waited until twenty-six weeks to start buying baby things. My mum made the process memorable by bringing me on a shopping trip to buy newborn vests, babygros, blankets and a beautiful little snowsuit to keep Sophia cosy in Kiev.

Like many would-be parents, we decided to totally upend our lives at this point by doing a lot of renovations on the house. There's something about a baby arriving that focuses the mind. Wes and I wanted to prepare our nest and be ready for the new person in our lives, and also to mark the transition between our lives as a couple and our lives as a family. I asked my friends what products did and didn't work for them and made a list, then we painted her nursery and Wes, who's handy at DIY, put together the cot, rocking chair and changing table we'd ordered online. Many people assume that this nesting behaviour is a hormonal response but I felt it so strongly with Sophia. I really embraced my nesting mode because it allowed me to mentally prepare for her arrival, as well as to take care of the practical side of things. I loved buying the tiny little outfits that she'd wear, carefully washing and folding them into her chest of drawers, imagining the little person who would soon fit into them. It was a very special time and I treasured it.

My wobbly moment came in early August, when the surrogate was about six months pregnant. I emailed the clinic's pregnancy coordinator and requested a picture of the baby bump to see what size it was. I told myself that this was just to reassure myself that everything was fine, but the idea of the human behind the pregnancy was definitely creeping into my mind. When I was sent a couple of full-length pictures of our surrogate, I gasped. Here was this beautiful smiling girl, with pink fingernails, standing against a pink wall, cradling her bump. I was overjoyed, but that feeling was overtaken by one of guilt and even envy. I couldn't carry my own child yet here was this woman living her life in a different country with our baby girl growing inside her. She'd be feeling those magical kicks and the weight of the baby in her womb. I began to wonder about her and what she did every day, what her partner and family thought about her choice to carry someone else's child, and what she felt about her bump. Suddenly, I found it hard to look at the photos because I desperately wanted to be her, to experience what she was experiencing. I was on the outside, looking in. I stared at them for a long time, crying tears of sadness for myself, despite the joy of seeing her growing tummy.

This is something that I really want people to know. While surrogacy is a wonderful and feasible route to parenthood for so many, there are other emotions that are more difficult to process – darker emotions that perhaps I hadn't anticipated or acknowledged. Now I understood why I hadn't explored the human side of the equation before. Of course, we'd been concerned that our surrogate would be healthy and feeling well, but now I'd crossed a boundary of some kind and had viewed the woman involved, rather than just the scan images of her uterus. It's natural, of course, but it brought up all sorts of uncomfortable feelings for me. I began to wonder if she was becoming attached to the baby growing inside her, but then realised that I couldn't continue to think like this. We had entered into the contract because we wanted a baby of our own and this woman had been generous enough to agree to give us the gift of life. I had to view the situation in this way for my own sanity. For that reason, I didn't ask for any more photos of the bump – it had brought up such difficult and unexpected emotions – but instead focused on moving forward to the thirty-week scan, then the next and the next after that until, at long last, the due date came into view.

CHAPTER 6

HOME FOR CHRISTMAS

When I woke on Saturday 5 October it was a bright, clear day and the morning sun was pouring in through the bedroom window. I was looking forward to a day of relaxing after the hectic last few months of house renovations, so when Wes suggested lunch in the Powerscourt Hotel, I readily agreed.

'Let's get dressed up and we'll make a nice afternoon of it,' he said. I was a bit puzzled because Wes never normally gives me outfit suggestions, but I put on a smart daytime dress and boots and off we went for our lunch. The sun was shining all the way, the Sugar Loaf looking so pretty in the distance. For the first time in a long while I could feel myself relax, looking forward to having a nice meal and hanging out with my husband, just feeling like a normal couple, taking our minds off the arrival of our baby in November.

I was slightly surprised when we arrived at the hotel and headed towards the elevators instead of to the restaurant at the back of the building. A member of staff greeted us and ushered us into the lift, pressing the button for the first floor. Where on earth were we going, I wondered. And when we emerged onto a corridor lined with doors, I couldn't help wondering if Wes had planned a surprise night away. Neither Wes nor the staff member said a word as we walked down the hallway, towards the set of double doors that opened into one of the meeting rooms. 'Here we are,' Wes said, opening the door. For a millisecond there was silence, followed by a yell of 'Surprise!' from a crowd of my dear friends and family. Shocked, I looked at Wes, but he nudged me gently inside the meeting room, which was festooned with balloons and confetti. A banner hanging across the ceiling said HAPPY BABY SHOWER. I couldn't believe it. I had no idea how Wes had managed to keep it from me, but it meant such a lot. A few of my friends had suggested it to him and he'd been delighted to be involved, happily agreeing to the subterfuge, inviting old school friends, cousins, my mum, my aunts, my closest friends. They'd put a lot of effort into planning the party and the room looked incredible. Sophia was given the most beautiful gifts and I really felt the love for her and support for us in the room. Of course, it wasn't the gifts that mattered to me, but the fact that my friends and family had put so much thought into the event, and I had most of the people who mattered in my life around me. *I may not have a baby bump*, I thought, *but I'm still going to be a mum and today we're all gathered here to celebrate it.* It was a very special afternoon.

It's funny looking back at that time because there was so much emotion and uncertainty attached to it. When I was pregnant with the twins, I found that I was much more laid-back and didn't experience the same extremes of highs and lows. As I said before, when you've had heartbreaks and losses, you begin to anticipate disaster and heartache all over again. It's hard to believe that things might go right for you. I think it also had to do with the fact that I wasn't carrying the baby myself. My child was developing in another woman thousands of miles away and I had no control over the outcome. All I could do was wait as patiently as I could and concentrate on gathering everything we'd need for our trip to Kiev in November for the birth.

Wes and I had asked the pregnancy coordinator if we might be present in the delivery room for Sophia's birth, but we both understood that this was entirely up to the surrogate. It was a lot to ask and we didn't want to overstep or invade her privacy. After all, we were strangers to her.

We'd celebrated Wes's birthday on 17 September and I'd flown to Lisbon with Mum and Dad for a short break afterwards. Dad was doing a couple of concerts over there, so I felt that joining them to support him and spend some time together would be a welcome distraction from planning for Kiev. We were sitting at breakfast in our hotel when my phone buzzed. It was an email from the pregnancy coordinator in Kiev with a long, comprehensive list of what we'd need to take with us in terms of baby equipment and clothing and recommendations for travel and apartments to rent adjacent to the maternity hospital. But the only part I saw were the words 'the surrogate is happy for you to be in the delivery room'. I broke down in tears and Mum looked at me in surprise across her coffee cup, saying, 'What's wrong with you?' I was sitting over my porridge, trying to conceal my sobs in the crowded restaurant, and just managing to get out the words, 'We're allowed to be in the room when the baby is being born.' Mum and Dad got emotional as well and the three of us sat in the hotel breakfast room crying happy tears. I was so grateful to our wonderful surrogate for allowing us this opportunity and for understanding that this was an important moment for us. It was such a generous offer and I was really touched.

Many people have asked me about the surrogate and what kind of connection we had with her. As I've said, we were careful to maintain boundaries for her sake as well as ours. On our side, there was probably a bit of fear involved that the surrogate might grow attached to the baby during her pregnancy – something that we've since found out is rare – but we were also conscious of not wanting to invade her privacy. I don't know if you necessarily do bond with a baby when you're pregnant, and I admittedly didn't bond with the twins closely throughout my pregnancy. To me, they were little passengers that I carefully carried and nurtured, but I did bond with them when they were born. Sometimes, I wonder if our surrogate felt a sadness parting with our baby when Sophia was born, but it's a delicate question and perhaps there is a part of me that doesn't want to fully know the answer.

We got the impression from the start that she was a very kind and sincere person, keeping us updated via the pregnancy coordinator on the pregnancy and reassuring us that she was feeling well. And even though I'd struggled initially with the idea of knowing her because it brought up so much emotion for me, I've since kept in touch with her, which has been another positive outcome of the surrogacy process. It's lovely to think that Sophia will have this tie to the country in which she was born and the woman who gave birth to her. I realise that she signed up for surrogacy not only for the financial benefits, because she had a child of her own to support, but also because she felt it would be an amazing gift to give to another couple. We will forever feel grateful to her.

As soon as I got the email from the clinic, I started to pack. I knew that we'd need warm clothes for winter-time in Kiev, as well as a baby car seat, clothes, sheets and blankets, bottles and our bottle steriliser. For Sophia's birth, we were keen to get everything organised well in advance just in case something happened and we needed to hop on a flight. Our surrogate had given birth to her own baby at thirty-eight weeks so we were advised by the doctor that she could arrive at any stage from thirty-seven weeks onwards, which would bring us to around the third week in November.

Mum popped over to our house when I was packing, watching me trying to stuff everything into a huge suitcase, and she couldn't help but laugh at me. 'How many times do you think she'll need to be changed in a day?' she said.

I replied, 'I don't know – I haven't a clue!' Like any prospective first-time parent, I was blissfully unaware of the work involved in caring for a newborn. I packed everything I could possibly think of, even though they have all the big baby brands in Kiev anyway, but for me, it was about preparing myself. It's the perfectionist in me, I suppose. In everything I do, whether it's an exam, a press conference or a cookery demonstration, I need to have the mental clarity of knowing that everything is prepared. Also, I think that if you are embarking on something new or daunting, doing everything you can to get yourself organised makes it less intimidating.

The fact that we'd be bringing our baby home for Christmas made it extra special for Wes and me. We felt like children again, getting excited about it all and imagining what our first Christmas might be like as a family. We had even decided on a name. In February of that year, when we'd been over for the egg-retrieval process, we'd gone out on a short amble the evening before my procedure to Saint Sophia's Cathedral, close to our hotel. It's a beautiful Byzantine architectural monument, painted green and white with those classic gold and green domes, and even though we're not religious, we felt very moved by the scale of it. We had both agreed that Sophia was a beautiful name, and if we had a daughter, calling her Sophia would be a poignant way to mark our journey in Kiev. When we found out in June that we were having a baby girl, we knew what we would call her. That connection to the city of her birth and our journey to having her felt important to us.

Even though we'd packed, we hadn't yet booked our flights. When you're waiting for a baby to be born, it's difficult to predict when it might happen. If we went over too early, we'd be hanging around, too late and we might even miss the birth, a thought we couldn't bear. Thankfully, the clinic came to the rescue by suggesting that we fly over on 11 November, when our surrogate would be thirty-seven weeks pregnant. It seemed auspicious because we'd signed the contracts on that same date the year before. There was a reassuring symmetry to it but it also made me realise just how lucky we were. To go from officially entering the surrogacy programme a year before to travelling to Kiev for the birth of our baby in less than a year was nothing short of a miracle. I'm aware that IVF sometimes needs two or three rounds to be successful, and even then, it's not guaranteed. From the beginning, I was conscious that we couldn't ask

or expect our surrogate to go through the process of injecting herself and preparing her womb over and over again
to accept an embryo, so I just felt this incredible sense of
gratitude that it had worked for us.

I made the practical arrangements for our trip well in advance,
renting a two-bedroom apartment near the hospital because
I knew we'd require more space and privacy than we'd find
in a hotel room, and we'd want to have our own kitchen and
washing machine for all those changes of baby clothes. The
second bedroom was for Mum, who was accompanying us
on the trip. She really wanted to be there for the birth of her
first grandchild, and it was important for us to have her there
because she's so experienced with babies and, having had
three of her own, she'd know exactly what to expect. I can
still remember telling her, 'I can't do this without you, Mum.
I don't know what I'm doing.' Never a truer word was said.

We arrived in Kiev on 11 November and spent the next
few days sorting out the baby equipment, setting up the
bottle-making machine, the steriliser, the changing table
and mat, the cot, the travel pram ... Wes was busy clicking
through videos on how to change a nappy and set up the
pram – thank goodness for YouTube. I was able to rent baby
equipment in Kiev quite easily, so I hired a bath, a weighing
scales and a cot. We were as ready as we'd ever be.

On the afternoon of 14 November, the clinic invited us
to the hospital for our surrogate's thirty-eight-week scan. It

was going to be the first time we'd meet her in person and it felt like a huge day for both of us. I made sure to pack tissues in my handbag because I had a feeling it would be an overwhelming experience. In normal life, I'm an emotionally stable adult, but I was so anxious throughout the pregnancy that towards the end I cried a lot of happy tears. We hopped in a cab to the maternity hospital, a brand new, modern building. The pregnancy coordinator was there to meet us and showed us to a small waiting area. Wes and I squeezed hands and waited to meet the woman who was carrying our child. I had a knot in my stomach and my heart was racing.

When the door opened, a petite and pretty young woman came in cradling her huge bump and smiled hello. My response was one of total shock. I'd thought about her daily for most of the year and seen the images of Sophia growing inside her; I'd even seen photos of her and had come to terms with it, although the images of this glowing young woman had stayed with me ever since. However, to be standing in front of her was surreal. I don't know how you can prepare yourself for an encounter like this. I don't honestly think you can. I just about managed to hold it together and the tissues remained in my handbag for the time being.

Even though she spoke little English and we needed a translator, I could see from her expression that she was probably more nervous of meeting us than we were of meeting her. But looking back, it was a much more relaxed occasion than Wes and I had anticipated. I'd expected all the complicated emotions I'd gone through to resurface, but they didn't. Over the previous couple of months, I had realised that I shouldn't be upset that someone else was experiencing 'my' pregnancy but just be appreciative instead. Although I couldn't take my eyes off her baby bump, I didn't feel any sense of jealousy or bitterness, just gratitude and excitement that we'd be meeting Sophia so soon.

We had a short chat then and asked her how she was feeling. She'd moved into the hospital for two weeks prior to the estimated birth date, which is standard procedure to enable the medical staff to monitor the pregnancy. A surrogate birth seems to be a detailed and well-planned operation. I loved that the clinic looked after them so well. I wouldn't have minded that when I was pregnant with the twins, moving into the hospital and putting my feet up!

The tissues came out when we went into the room for the scan. We settled down on chairs beside the examination bed as the doctor placed the Doppler monitor on the bump to check the baby's heartbeat, and soon it rang out in the little room, loud and clear. I started to cry. I couldn't believe that I was hearing my baby's heartbeat for the very first time – that her birth was real and would be happening any day now. It was almost too much to take in. Our surrogate said, via the translator, that she felt it wouldn't be too long, possibly within the next week, because she'd started to feel some cramping. Then the tears really began to flow. In a week's time, we'd be a family.

While we were waiting, Mum and Wes and I spent an enjoyable ten days continuing to explore Kiev, a city we were beginning to know pretty well at this stage. As we'd pass a particular favourite restaurant or café, the staff would wave at us and say 'Hi!' We felt very much at home and we're grateful to have such happy memories of Sophia's birthplace. Every night at our evening meal we'd have a guess about what day she'd arrive, but as the days passed, we began to wonder if our surrogate had been right. On Wednesday 20 November, we went out for dinner at a Thai restaurant and at the end, as usual, we speculated. Mum said, 'It's going to happen tomorrow, I'm telling you!'

I said, 'No, it'll be Friday, I'm sure of it.' Why had I forgotten that mums are always right? The next morning, Mum and Wes got breakfast ready while I had a shower. When I stepped out and checked my phone, I found a series of missed calls from the pregnancy coordinator and then a text: *She's in labour, contractions every 60 seconds, you need to get to the hospital immediately.* I yelled, 'Everyone, the baby is on her way, let's get going!' There was a scramble for clothes and our hospital bags and we were out the door in fifteen minutes. Mum grabbed some snacks for breakfast, we popped the car seat into the back of the waiting taxi and then we set off to the hospital to finally meet our daughter. The atmosphere in the cab was almost festive as the streets of the city whizzed by. I looked at the people thronging the pavements, on their way to work or shopping, and thought,

In just a few hours I'll become a mum and my life will change forever.

The panic subsided when we reached the hospital and met the pregnancy coordinator, who was in constant contact with the doctor and reassured us that we still had a bit of time to get settled in before Sophia arrived. We were brought to our room, which was a little suite with a bedroom, sitting room and bathroom, and kept ourselves occupied by lining Sophia's cot with a fresh sheet and arranging neat piles of tiny newborn nappies on the changing table. My hands were shaking with excitement. I even had a few extra minutes to dry my hair and spruce myself up a bit. I can remember thinking, *I'm going to meet my daughter so I should probably make an effort!* After about an hour, the doctor told us it was time to come up to the birthing room. We were handed blue scrubs, theatre caps and shoe covers, and we carefully washed our hands before being brought upstairs. As the lift ascended to the third floor, my heart was thumping and my head was spinning with nervous anticipation. Wes and I couldn't stop grinning at each other as he squeezed my hand.

We were asked to wait outside the room for a moment, and then the door opened to the surrogate in a birthing chair, deeply concentrating as she gave birth to our baby. I froze at the door and Mum gave me a nudge, saying 'Go, go!' and urged me inside. It was all very focused as our surrogate pushed hard and Sophia's head appeared, while the doctor prepared to gently turn her shoulders. It felt bizarre to witness something so private and intimate as our child being born. I stood there, unsure where to put myself or how to deal with what I was seeing. A stranger was giving birth, but to our child, and I didn't know how to react. Nobody gives you a manual for situations like this.

Then, with one more push, out Sophia came, a little pink-ish-blue doll with a scrunched-up face, crying hysterically at the shock of being born. The doctor gently turned her around to face us and asked me if I'd like to cut the umbilical cord, at our surrogate's suggestion. The only thing I could think of to say was, 'I'm left-handed, is that OK?' Honestly, I felt so silly, but the doctor just laughed and said, 'Of course, it's fine.' As I cut her cord, it felt like such a special and symbolic moment, breaking the bond between Sophia and the surrogate and giving her to us, her mum and dad. Wiping tears from his eyes, Wes gave me a huge hug.

I was so overwhelmed that my mind was a complete blank as Sophia was taken by one of the nurses to be cleaned and wrapped. I turned to the doctor and said, 'Is she OK? Is everything OK?' He smiled warmly and gave me a hug and said, 'Everything's fine. She's healthy.' At this point, relief and the breathtaking emotion of the moment hit me and I burst into tears. In between sobs, all I could think of to say to the woman lying there, exhausted, was, 'Thank you, thank you, thank you.' I must have said it twenty times but she didn't have the energy to reply. It had been a quick labour, but an intense one, and she was clearly worn out.

It was hard to believe that she had gone through all of this for us.

I didn't want to let Sophia out of my sight, so we followed the nurse into the adjacent room, where they weighed and measured her. She was 6lb 9oz, healthy and proportionate. I'm sure every parent thinks this, but to me and to Wes she was absolutely perfect. We admired her tiny fingers and toes, then I was asked to lie on a chair to snuggle her to my chest. I'd worn a button-down top with a vest underneath and Sophia was wrapped up with a little hat on her head and laid gently on my chest. That skin-to-skin contact was wonderful. I'll never forget it. After a while Wes held her too, cradling her in his arms and telling her that she was beautiful, but at that stage, Sophia was getting hungry and began to scrabble towards Wes's nipple. All she got for her trouble was a mouthful of chest hair!

From the moment we'd been handed Sophia, she was ours, which was scary and exhilarating at the same time. While the surrogate was monitored and given a chance to rest, we returned to our little suite with our newborn to begin our new lives as Mum and Dad. It felt surreal knowing that we were officially parents and totally responsible for this new life, a real journey into the unknown. Thankfully, the nurses stayed for a while to show us how much milk to give her – just a tiny amount at first – and how to put on her nappy. Feeding her was an amazing experience – watching her drink milk for the first time. I was impressed by the strength of her sucking reflex, an important mammalian survival instinct, but after a little while she got very tired and nodded off. The room became silent as we all tried to assimilate the events of the previous few hours. I looked at my daughter sleeping in her little cot and said, 'Is she real? Did that just happen today?'

Our first night with Sophia felt like a strange dream, with me watching her like a hawk, making sure she was breathing, and setting my alarm for every two-and-a-half hours because she needed to be woken for feeds. I managed to fall asleep at 6 a.m. for a couple of hours, before the nurses came in to check on us. Sophia developed a bit of jaundice the next day, as is common in newborns, so she had twenty-four hours of phototherapy under a bili-light lamp in our room.

Being a first-time mum, I wanted to do everything right and enjoy the experience as much as possible. I bought a notebook to note her feeding times and how many wet and dirty nappies she produced, so I could monitor Sophia's development. Those of you who have been newbie parents will relate to all the questions that go through your mind when a baby is crying. Is she hungry? Has she got wind? Is her nappy dirty? Is she hot/cold? The questions were endless and the answers not always that obvious. Wes and I were guided by Mum, thankfully, but it was still all down to us. The thought of being responsible for the life of this tiny person was daunting and exciting at the same time.

On our third day in the hospital, as we were packing up to leave, there was a gentle knocking on our door and the surrogate arrived to meet Sophia for the first time. I thought it might have been a little awkward, but it wasn't. She leaned into Sophia's cot and looked at her and said, 'Oh, she's beautiful. Congratulations.' This wonderful woman had just given birth to our baby yet was congratulating us – it seemed strange, but she didn't seem to be uncomfortable with the situation. I was pleased that she'd come to visit because I really wanted her to meet the baby to whom she'd given birth, and I also needed to say thank you again, even though words didn't seem adequate to express our gratitude to her. She had been so relaxed and generous to us – I wondered how she felt about this final parting from the baby. She said she was looking forward to returning to her hometown to rest and spend time with her daughter and partner, whom she hadn't seen in the past couple of weeks.

Then we zipped Sophia up in her cosy snowsuit against the biting winter cold and brought her back to the apartment. We may have been many miles from Dublin but bringing her across the threshold still felt like bringing her home. She was ours.

Back at the apartment, we arranged to chat to a paediatrician to ask all the questions we needed about Sophia – and there were many. A friend who had also gone through surrogacy in Kiev recommended a paediatric doctor with excellent English, who called to the apartment the next day. She checked Sophia over, pronounced her healthy and well and we bombarded her with questions. How could we keep her umbilical cord clean? Did we need to give her vitamin D drops? Could we take her outside? The poor woman must have wondered if we had ever seen a baby in our lives, but she answered our queries thoroughly. Yes, we could take her out if she was well wrapped up, and so, for the next few days, our big outing was to the park across the road, pushing Sophia in her pram. Timing was of the essence: we had to make sure that she was fed and changed and we were fed and changed out of our pyjamas too!

Of course, we were nervous at the beginning. The paediatrician had told us that babies are more robust than you might think, but we couldn't believe that this tiny person might one day grow into a healthy little girl. She looked so fragile and delicate. We adapted and learned quickly, though, thanks to our two weeks of 'baby bootcamp'. Mum was teaching us everything she knew and it was a great help. Even though we were a bit isolated, with just the three of us in the apartment in Kiev, it was lovely to have that uninterrupted time together, without visitors or distractions, to get to know Sophia and focus fully on her every need.

This was something of a relief because Sophia was quite colicky at the beginning, and we became severely sleep-deprived. We regularly sat down for breakfast at two or three o'clock in the afternoon because we'd been up all night soothing her, and even though we were overjoyed, we were still relentlessly exhausted. It felt like constant jet lag. Sometimes, I'd hit a wall and wonder, how can I continue?

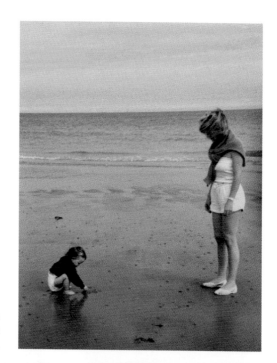

Playing in the sand with Mum at Ballyhealy Beach in Wexford, summer 1985.

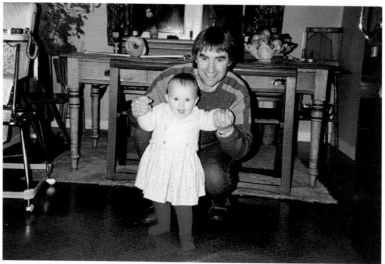

With my dad at our family home in Dublin, February 1985.

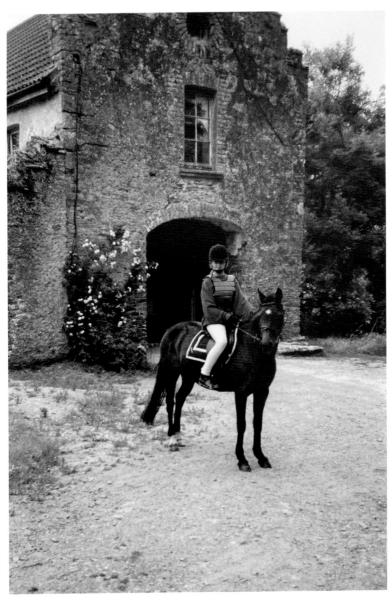

Riding Molly in front of the old brick coach-house at Bargy Castle in
spring 1996.

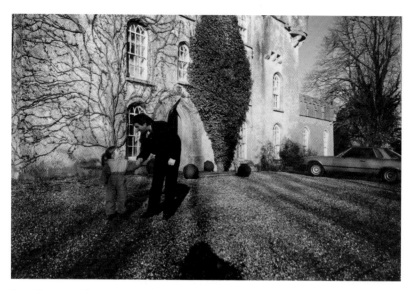

Standing outside Bargy Castle with my dad, winter 1986.

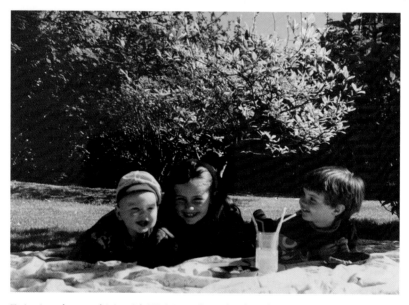

Enjoying the sunshine with Hubie and Michael in the garden at our family home in Dalkey, Co. Dublin, during summer 1991.

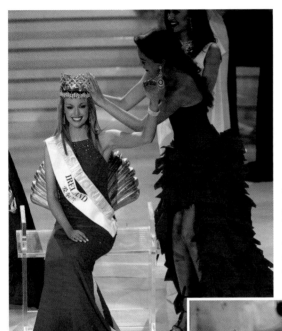

The crowning moment of Miss World 2003 by the 2002 winner, Azra Akin. (© *REUTERS / Alamy Stock Photo*)

Waving to the audience as Miss World 2003 in the Crown of Beauty Theatre, in the tropical city of Sanya, Hainan Island, China. (© *Frederick J. Brown, AFP/Getty Images*)

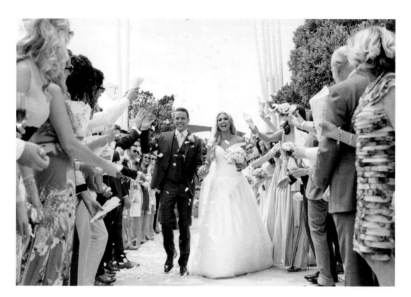

Wedding day confetti and celebrations with family and friends after our marriage ceremony in Ibiza, on 1 June 2014.

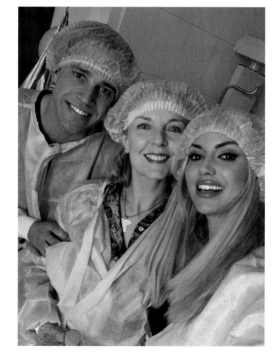

A quick photo with Mum and Wes in our scrubs on 21 November 2019 in the maternity hospital in Kiev, just minutes before Sophia was born.

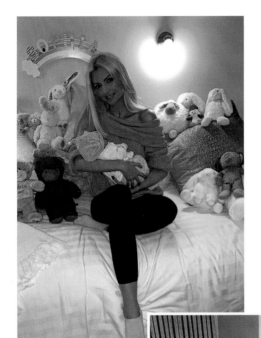

Sitting amongst the numerous cuddly toys in Sophia's nursery in December 2019. She was just four-and-a-half weeks old.

A special moment introducing Sophia to her great-grand-mother, Maeve Davison, in Bargy Castle in late December 2019.

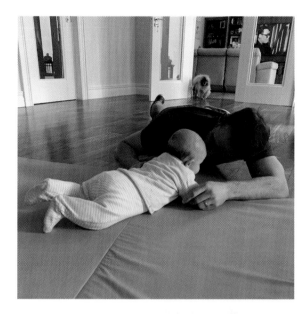

Wes and Sophia at home in March 2020, during the first lockdown of the pandemic.

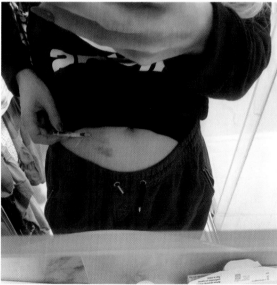

I took this on 10 May 2020. I was seven weeks pregnant with Hugo and Oscar and had to inject my stomach daily with heparin to reduce the risk of developing a blood clot.

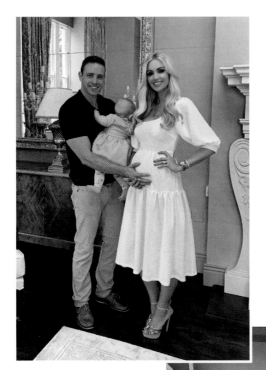

This photo with Wes and Sophia was taken by his mum in July 2020 to accompany our pregnancy announcement on Instagram. I was almost 19 weeks pregnant with the twins.

Prenatal training with Jessica Kavanagh at Inform Fitness in October 2020. I was just over 28 weeks pregnant, and I enjoyed working out three times a week throughout my pregnancy.

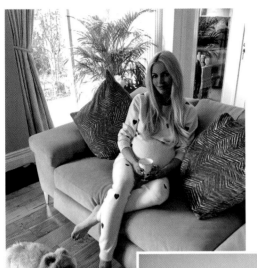

October 2020. I had
to spend a lot of time
relaxing on the sofa
once the third trimester
arrived!

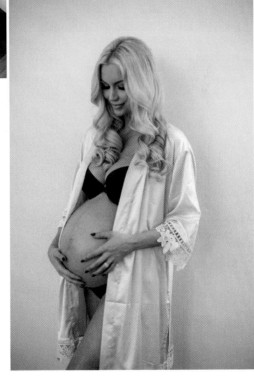

Admiring my twin
baby bump at 32
weeks pregnant in
late October 2020.
(*Courtesy of Lili
Forberg*)

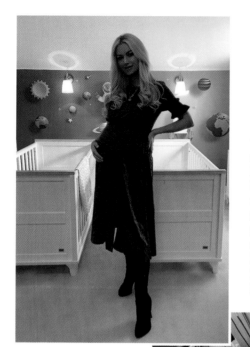

17 November 2020. I was so proud of the nursery we had designed for the boys, based on an outer-space theme. I was about to drive into Dublin city centre to go to my final scan, but ended up spending that night in hospital. The twins were born less than 24 hours later.

Lying on my bed in the National Maternity Hospital on 17 November 2020, the night before Hugo and Oscar were born, as their heart rates were monitored by a midwife. This is the final photo I took of my baby bump.

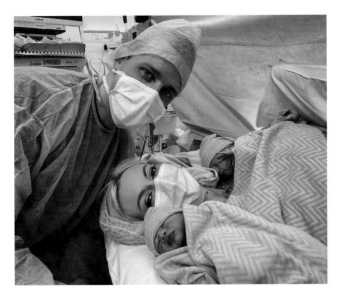

Moments after Hugo and Oscar were born by C-section on 18 November 2020. This was our birth announcement photo and an incredibly proud, exciting moment for our new family of five.

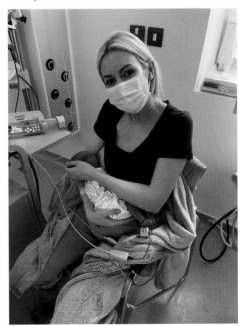

A proud moment breastfeeding Hugo for the first time on 21 November 2020 in the neonatal department at the National Maternity Hospital, Holles Street.

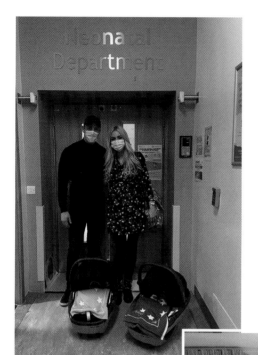

Wes and I leaving the neonatal department for the final time on 25 November 2020 to bring our boys home to meet their sister and grandparents. It was a very emotional moment.

Christmas Eve 2020 with Hugo and Oscar, who were just five weeks old.

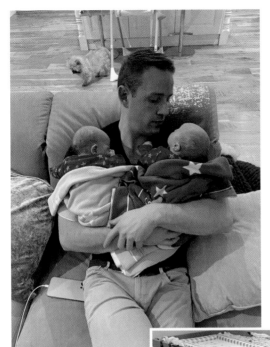

Wes cuddling the twins at home on Christmas Day 2020.

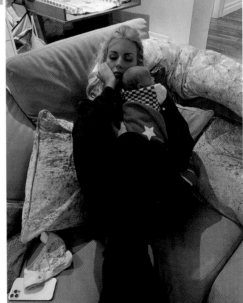

St. Stephen's Day 2020, feeling exhausted after our Christmas Day celebrations and taking a short nap with Hugo on our sofa at home.

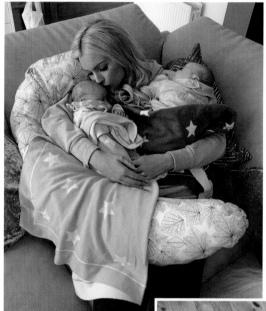

Cuddles on the sofa
with the boys in
early January 2021.

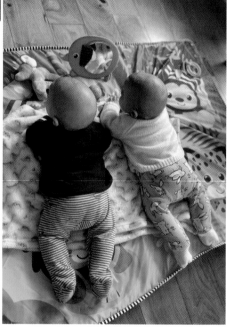

The boys enjoying
'tummy time' on their
play-mat in early March
2021.

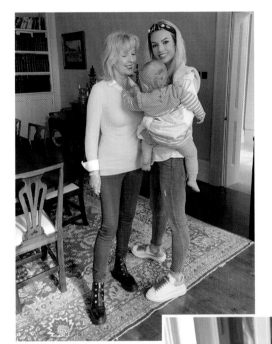

Enjoying Mother's Day 2021 with Sophia and Mum at my parents' home in Co. Wicklow.

Introducing my grandmother, Maeve Davison, to the twins for the first time. Pictured with Hugo at our home in Dublin, May 2021.

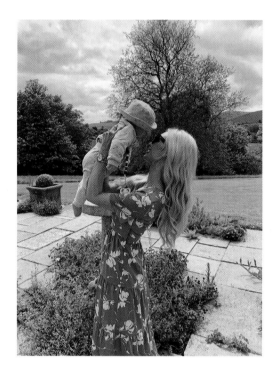

Enjoying a sunny day with Oscar in the garden of the family home in Enniskerry, Co. Wicklow, May 2021.

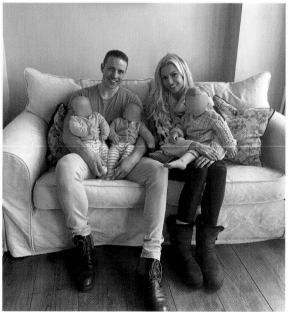

Enjoying life as a family of five, March 2021.

I now know that feeling a bit desperate is part of having a newborn baby. When you are sleep-deprived, you can lose all sense of perspective, and it can have a negative impact on your mental health. Anytime I'd start to feel sorry for myself, I would remember that this was what I had wished for and everything is just a fleeting moment in time. In fact, one of the best pieces of advice I was given was 'Everything is a phase and it will pass.' It's so true. With a baby, everything is a first: the first smiles and giggles, the first taste of solid food, the first word, the first steps, and then it's on to the next phase in their development. I found that I had to live in the moment with Sophia and be mindful of the present because it's difficult to plan too far ahead with babies. I really like that.

The legal process that parents through surrogacy follow is that the Irish father applies to the court for a Declaration of Parentage, Guardianship Order and Custody Order. An order dispenses with the necessity to seek the consent of the surrogate mother to the issuance of an Irish passport for the child. Once those orders are granted, the Irish father (now guardian) can apply for his child's Irish passport. Wesley and I, with our solicitor Annette Hickey, followed that legal process. In Ireland, the Irish mother can apply for a guardianship order when she has shared the day-to-day responsibility for caring for the child for two years.

Saturday 7 December was the day we brought our baby girl home for Christmas. After the morning spent hastily packing up everything from the apartment, between feeds and changes, and dashing to the airport, I remember standing on the tarmac at the bottom of the steps, surrounded by all her baby paraphernalia. I'd spoken to a lot of friends with babies about how they managed to travel and had picked up a few tips: I was able to zip her car seat into a protective travel bag and get it onto the plane with my luggage, and I'd brought a travel pushchair that could be folded and put into an overhead locker. I had her carefully packed changing bag with me so I could feed her during the flight and change her nappy. She slept almost all the way home, oblivious to the magnitude of the journey for us.

Landing in Dublin, we were amazed to see Christmas decorations everywhere and hear the merry songs playing through the loudspeakers. In Kiev there had been no real festive atmosphere, so it was comforting and nostalgic to experience it in the airport. As we walked into the arrivals area and spotted Dad waiting for us, it felt as if Christmas had come early. He'd only finished his European concert tour a couple of days before and hadn't been able to join us in Kiev, so watching him meet his granddaughter for the first time was a memorable moment. He cradled her in his arms, gazing in amazement at her peaceful sleeping face.

We tucked Sophia up under a fleecy blanket in her car seat in the back of Dad's car, with me sitting beside her. It was hard to believe that we were finally back in Ireland with our precious baby. I imagine it's the same for any new parent coming home: that sense of nervous excitement and the feeling of embarking on a whole new phase of life – there was no difference to me because she was born through surrogacy. And the welcome home we were given was exactly the same too, with Wes's family there to greet us, having decorated the house with pink banners, balloons and bunches of fresh flowers. Recently, I came across a video that Wes made of us taking Sophia on her first-ever tour of her new home. She was still fast asleep as we carried her from room to room, telling her, 'That's Mummy and Daddy's room, where you'll be sleeping, and there's your room, where you'll sleep when you're older, and there's the rocking chair and the cot ...' It didn't matter that she wasn't aware of any of it – to us, the feelings were indescribable. Finally, we did it, I thought. We actually did it.

CHAPTER 7

A GLIMMER OF HOPE

When we were waiting for Sophia to arrive in 2019, I remember saying to Mum, 'It'll be brilliant to take her everywhere with us and include her in everything we do. She'll just slot into our lives so well.'

Mum had nearly fallen over laughing. 'Rosie,' she said. 'You have no idea. You'll see when she's born.' How right she was! The next few weeks after our return were a blur of late nights, early mornings, constant feeds, piles of laundry and lots of excited visitors. We used to joke that Sophia was a party animal: she slept all day and stayed awake all night, which I was assured is normal in the early months before any kind of differentiation between day and night is made, but it was also exhausting. Wes had returned to work when we got home, because Christmas is a really busy time in his business, and even though my mum and his mum were on hand to help, I really tried to do everything myself. As tired as I'd get, I wanted to have that feeling of totally being her mum because I still felt a deep, lingering guilt that I hadn't been able to carry her myself and give birth to her.

I'm not going to sugar-coat the situation. It was really tough. Some nights, Sophia wouldn't go to sleep until seven o'clock in the morning, then she'd wake a few hours later for her next feed and I'd get her up, change her and make us both presentable for visitors, even though I could barely open my eyes. I wanted to show that I had everything under control, which amuses me now. No new mother is 'in control'. It was an exhausting and intense battle of emotions. Every day I'd feel thankful and happy but oh-so tired! I dreamed about having a sleep-in. Of course, as soon as I even thought about complaining, I'd remind myself just how much we'd longed for Sophia and then I'd feel guilty. As a new mum, I think it's hard to get the balance right, and guilt can be very much part of the experience. Every day is a learning process, as you get to know this new little human. I gratefully accepted guidance from close friends and family, but I tried my best to block out a lot of the unsolicited advice that comes with having a newborn. It's mostly well-meaning, but having too much information and instruction can be overwhelming. The best advice I can offer to new parents is get to know your own baby, don't compare yourself or your parenting skills to others' and trust your instincts.

I don't know what I'd have done without Wes. I used to jokingly call him the Angel of the Night when he'd arrive into our bedroom at four o'clock in the morning from the spare room, where he was sleeping to get some rest ahead of a busy day at work, because he'd have heard Sophia crying. One night when he came in, Sophia was in her cot bawling and I was in the bed beside her sobbing too. 'I can't do this,' I wept. 'I'm too tired!' Wes came to the rescue, picking up Sophia to change her, feed her and soothe her back to sleep while I managed to nod off. Sleep deprivation is one of the worst forms of torture, I think.

Sophia was by no means a 'problem' baby. During the day she was happy and always smiling, but she suffered regularly with symptoms of colic in the early months, and as any new parent will tell you, there's not an awful lot you can do about it. We changed her formula, gave her lactase enzyme drops and simethicone and sought advice from my GP and the district nurse. But she still suffered, particularly in the evenings, and we spent hours gently rocking her. They often call this period the 'fourth trimester', when babies' immature digestive systems are still developing and patience is really the only solution. In the meantime, Wes and I shared the parenting jobs. He would come home from work tired, I'd hand Sophia over to him and go upstairs for a short nap. Then I'd take her and he'd go for a snooze and, somehow, we managed to cope and stay relatively sane. We've always worked well as a team.

Christmas in my parents' home in Enniskerry provided a welcome break from the routine, although I'm always amazed at how much you need for an overnight stay with a baby. We piled her travel cot, milk machine, steriliser, bottles, blankets, changes of clothes, nappies, wipes and our own bags into the car and set off on the short drive from our house. It felt like the most magical Christmas being there with our family and new baby. On St Stephen's Day, we packed everything up again and went to Wes's home for a second Christmas dinner, grateful that our two families had managed to spend the festive season with Sophia. In spite of the tiredness, it was such an enjoyable few days. I can remember looking around at everyone tucking into Christmas dinner and feeling blissfully happy that I had my family. I felt an enormous sense of gratitude for our good fortune and thought back to the time when Wes and I had spoken about what life might be like without children in it. He'd reassured me that we'd be happy and live purposeful lives packed with travel, friends and fun. Life doesn't stop being meaningful because you don't have children, but our happiness was complete with Sophia in it. And my powerful biological desire to care for and nurture a baby of my own had been satisfied.

I had kept in touch with our surrogate after the birth and she sent me a sweet message when Sophia was a month old, on 21 December: 'Happy one month to Sophia. Hope you have a lovely Christmas.' It meant a lot to me that she had kept us in her thoughts.

Despite the sleepless nights and sometimes difficult days, Wes and I hadn't forgotten our wish to have a second child, a sibling for Sophia. I grew up with two brothers and knew that I always wanted two or even three children. We'd been so impressed with our surrogate throughout the entire process, and found her so positive and gentle, that I'd mentioned in passing to our pregnancy coordinator that we would love for her to carry our child again in the future.

On New Year's Day 2020, we'd organised a family photoshoot at home with a photographer friend of mine. The photos were just for us and for close family to celebrate Sophia's arrival, and he took some lovely shots. I'm so glad we have them to remember Sophia's early days as a tiny baby.

The photographer had just gone home and we were tidying up the makeshift studio when my phone beeped with a message from the surrogate: 'I want to wish you a very Happy New Year and I'd like to let you know that I would love to give Sophia a sibling. I've decided that I want to give your family another baby.' I could feel tears welling up as Wes asked me what on earth had happened. Wordlessly, I showed him the message we'd both hoped to receive. We were ecstatic and relieved. We'd been nervous about the clinic having to begin the search for a different surrogate,

of sleep overnight. Wes and I finally managed to get five or six hours of unbroken sleep a night, which you can seemingly adapt to and survive on. However, I couldn't shake the feeling of heavy exhaustion that had been hanging over me for a month or so, and even the thought of certain foods made me feel a bit queasy. One night, Wes had ordered an Indian takeaway and asked if I wanted some and I said, 'Oh no, even the smell is making me feel sick.' I assumed that the few months of sleep deprivation and adapting to life as a mum was affecting my body in various unpredictable ways. Then my brother and his girlfriend flew to Tulum on holiday and kept sending us photos of their colourful Mexican meals and all the fresh avocados they were enjoying. All I could think about was eating Mexican food. I had these intense cravings, especially when I was up in the night feeding Sophia. I'd go to the supermarket and eye up the taco kits on the shelves, drooling over the images on the front of the boxes. I made a huge bowl of guacamole one day and polished off the lot. Another evening, Wes wandered into the room eating a bowl of cereal with ice-cold oat milk. I asked him for a spoonful and it seemed like the most delicious food I'd ever tasted! I figured it was all down to my inconsistent eating habits when Sophia had first arrived. I'd eaten anything that was put in front of me or nothing at all. Spending all day at home with her, changing her nappy and feeding her every few hours, it would sometimes get to five o'clock and I'd realise that I'd had nothing all day except coffee. I put my symptoms down to exhaustion and lack of proper nutrition and resolved to start taking some supplements and eating a more balanced diet.

I didn't take maternity leave when Sophia arrived, so I returned to work in January. I relied on my mum a lot to help out as we didn't have childcare and she often took Sophia to her house for the day when I was working. I had a number of events and an overnight trip to Germany planned for early February. I really missed Sophia, of course, but I found that I quite enjoyed the time away and a long, uninterrupted sleep in my hotel bed. In the third week of February, I was booked for a photo shoot for TanOrganic to promote a new tanning range, for which I was asked to wear a pair of white shorts and a bikini top. Normally this wouldn't have bothered me because it's the most effective way to demonstrate how their products look, but my shorts felt alarmingly tight. I remember saying to the PR girl, 'I'm sorry, I feel really bloated today – it must be that time of the month.' And then it suddenly occurred to me that I hadn't had a period since December. That must be it, I thought. All the stress and lost sleep of being a new mum had clearly had an impact on my body's hormones.

Later that week, my brain fog began to lift, and by the end of February, I was feeling mentally clearer and physically more energetic, as the tiredness and nausea had disappeared. I remember thinking that it was fortunate timing because I was due on the *Late Late Show* on 28 February to talk about our fertility struggles and surrogacy journey. They had been in touch with me to appear on the show in autumn 2019, but I didn't feel that the timing was right because Sophia hadn't yet been born and therefore our story hadn't reached its conclusion. Now that it had, I should have felt excited to share it with everyone. Instead, about two weeks before the interview I remember thinking that I couldn't possibly appear live on national television to discuss something so personal. How could I get through it without crying? I'll make a fool of myself, I thought. I wasn't sure if I had the emotional strength for it.

Thankfully, Wes talked me into it. 'Think of all the people who are going through what we went through,' he said. 'They're probably feeling alone right now, and your story could really help.' He was right, of course. I summoned up all of my courage and did the interview with Ryan Tubridy, who was kind and encouraging. I couldn't believe the out-pouring of love and support from the viewers. Even more importantly, the interview received an overwhelmingly posi-tive response from people who were struggling through their own fertility issues. I was so glad I'd done it. It was the kind of story I would have found inspiring to hear when Wes and I were enduring our repeat pregnancy losses, so the feedback meant a lot to me.

The compassion shown to us was a huge boost, and since life with Sophia had settled down to a more predict-able pattern, I had started going back to the gym, cooking homemade meals and beginning to feel like myself again. Funnily enough, my long-awaited period seemed to arrive on Saturday 29 February. There was a little light patchy bleeding, but I put this down to my body recalibrating after the stress of the last few months, and it continued like that for a couple of days. I thought nothing of it. On Tuesday of that week, I was getting Sophia ready for bed on her changing table in the kitchen when I felt a sudden, intense cramping. 'Wes,' I called. 'Can you finish changing Sophia? I'm having really bad cramps. I need to sit down for a minute.'

I shuffled over to the sofa, leaning over the back of it to ease the pain in my abdomen. 'Ouch, this is bad,' I said. 'Wes, would you mind filling a hot-water bottle for me?' He obliged once he'd changed Sophia, and I lay down on the sofa for a few minutes, the hot-water bottle on my tummy. The intense cramping wasn't easing. In fact, it was getting worse. I was feeling quite faint and shaky with the pain. 'I need to go to the bathroom,' I said suddenly. I stood up and felt a gush of warmth between my legs. Pulling down my leggings, I saw a stream of fresh blood followed by two huge clots the size of the palm of my hand. Wes and I stood there in shock, staring at the floor. 'I think it's just my period,' I said doubtfully. 'I haven't had one in a couple of months, so maybe that's why it's so heavy.' Wes ran off to get a mop and disinfectant and I went to the bathroom to sit down for a second. When I shakily stood up again, another couple of clots came out. I felt myself breaking out in a cold, queasy sweat, staring in horror at the bathroom tiles covered in blood. It looked as though a murder had taken place.

Wes appeared at the door. 'Are you OK?' he asked, surveying the scene in the bathroom. I could see the look of panic in his eyes and I didn't want to worry him, so I replied, 'I'm fine, honestly, it's just a heavy period.'

He looked doubtful. 'I'm not happy with the blood you're losing. I'm calling your mum.'

'No, it's fine,' I protested. But there was blood all over my hands and legs, smears across the toilet and puddles on the floor, so when he insisted, I didn't argue. Feeling weak and dizzy, I lay down on the bath mat and listened to Wes on the phone to Mum. 'Hi, Diane. I think you should come over. Rosie's losing blood and I don't know what's happening.' My poor mum must have got a terrible fright, but of course she came straight to our house, took one look at me and said, 'I'm going to bring you to Holles Street.' Wes had shown her the blood clots and an odd piece of liverish tissue that had emerged from me, and even though she was trying not to look too worried, I could tell that she was concerned. By this point, I was shivering, so Wes wrapped my bathrobe around my shoulders while Mum found a pair of runners and a warm coat to put on me. 'Do you have any pads you can wear on the way in?' she asked.

'I don't think so.' I hadn't bothered to buy any because of the lack of period over the past few months, so Mum grabbed a couple of Sophia's nappies. 'Here,' she said, handing me one.

'You'll have to use this.' I was past caring at that point as I stuffed it into my leggings and slid another into my coat pocket. Mum and Wes helped me into her car and she drove us to the hospital.

We were taken quickly into the emergency room, and once she had checked my temperature and blood pressure, the nurse asked me if I had been pregnant.

'Oh, no,' I replied confidently. 'It was just a heavy period.' I was absolutely convinced of it. After all, what else could it be?

They did a urine pregnancy test and took some tissue samples from me, which were sent to the lab. After a little while, the nurse came back and said, 'Well, you actually were pregnant. We've just got a positive confirmation from your pregnancy test and the tissue sample examined in the lab was positive for pregnancy. When was your last period?'

I could barely take it all in. None of it made sense. I thought about it for a few seconds and answered, '19 December.' We counted back and she said, 'That would have made you ten-and-a-half weeks pregnant.' There was a short pause while I said nothing at all, and then she added, 'I'm so sorry. Is there anything we can do for you?'

'This is amazing,' I said, smiling broadly. 'I've never got this far in a pregnancy.' She looked startled at my excited response, but that was my reaction. Of course, I was in shock at experiencing my fifteenth miscarriage, but I was also astonished that I'd been pregnant and hadn't realised.

I'd gone into the hospital in total denial and now I was faced with the reality that my body had achieved something it had never been able to do before – progress a pregnancy past six-and-a-half weeks.

The nurse brought me tea and a couple of slices of toast with jam and gently informed me that they offered a counselling service if I would like to be referred. My reply probably surprised her a bit. 'Thank you but I have a three-month-old to go home to. I didn't even know I was pregnant. I'm perfectly fine,' I insisted. And it was true, in a way. With every previous pregnancy, I'd been so aware of it, my every cell tuned into the fact that I was pregnant, but once Sophia had been born and we'd been given that lovely news from our surrogate in early January, I'd stopped thinking about it. In my mind, our family would be complete. Our surrogate would be giving us our much-wanted children and I wouldn't be carrying them because I believed I was medically incapable of it. Now, though, a tiny doubt began to creep into my mind. Could there be a chance that I might? Interestingly, both the doctor and nurse had said to me separately that night that I would be 'very fertile' after a ten-week miscarriage and to 'be careful' if I wanted to avoid another pregnancy so soon.

When I looked back over the previous few months, I worked out that we must have conceived around 1 or 2 January. My memory was fuzzy and Wes and I couldn't quite work out how it had happened with the sleep deprivation.

But it obviously had. So much made sense now. I'd been popping out to the supermarket to buy an array of foods to satisfy my cravings and there was the strange nausea and tiredness. I was amazed that I'd been looking after a new-born while in the early stages of pregnancy. I had appeared on the *Late Late Show* to speak about not being able to have a baby while I was actually almost ten weeks pregnant. The irony.

It was a big shock physically, and it took me a few days to recover from the blood loss and tiredness, but it didn't have the same emotional effect on me as my previous pregnancy losses. I was philosophical, in a way, while the scientist in me was curious about how differently my body had behaved this time. I wondered why my body had allowed pregnancy tissue to develop. I suppose the answer could be obvious in one way: we had stopped trying to have a baby ourselves and I had also slowed down with Sophia, adapting my life to her sleeping and feeding schedule. I wasn't racing around the place from one meeting or work obligation to the other. Maybe I'd simply let go and allowed my body to heal.

In hindsight, it's easy to rationalise, to tell myself what so many people had told me: that I needed to do less and to slow down. I'd describe my lifestyle up until Sophia was born as fast-paced and I was always on display. I made sure that I had a busy schedule, probably to distract myself from the reality that I wasn't able to have a family, ironically. You don't realise how much you're pushing yourself until you look back. Now I wonder if maybe my pregnancy had been a little nudge from my body to tell me that tuning into it a little bit more and reducing my stress levels might be part of the answer.

It was almost 1 a.m. by the time I was discharged from Holles Street that night, and I felt so grateful to get home to Sophia, fast asleep in her cot beside our bed. If we didn't have her, the miscarriage would have absolutely devastated me. But I couldn't shake the memory of that pregnancy. Could it be that I might be able to have a baby after all? I wondered. Was there a glimmer of hope that something might have changed within me? After all, we'd heard miracle stories of couples who had been trying for years without success and suddenly it had worked. Maybe that could happen to us. It had been a long time since we'd been actively trying for a baby. I wondered if I was up to the worry and stress that might result, and I really didn't want to go through yet another miscarriage. But I also didn't want to give up trying if there was even a tiny chance it might happen. Maybe we wouldn't actively try, but nor would we not try. To be perfectly honest, I never made an effort to prevent it. When you've been through a battle with infertility, you might be bruised and battered, but you never fully give up hope.

And then, in March 2020, Covid happened and changed our lives for ever.

CHAPTER 8

WE MADE A WISH AND TWO CAME TRUE

After I had recovered from the shock pregnancy and miscarriage, I put them to the back of my mind, mainly because I was finding it difficult to process my feelings about them. I wondered if the foetus at one stage had a heartbeat. What caused it to fail? There were so many unanswered questions. I hadn't had the chance to think about it, to calculate a due date and to daydream about what I might call the baby. I thought back to all the places I'd been and people I'd seen over the past couple of months, unknowingly with a tiny baby growing inside me.

I was trying to protect myself emotionally too. I vividly remember the night we drove home from the hospital, telling Mum that I had a photo shoot for a magazine the next morning. I had thought about cancelling but didn't want to let the team down. Thankfully, Mum put me straight. 'Go to a photo shoot at eight o'clock in the morning – are you mad? You've lost all that blood, you're exhausted, I found you lying on the floor tonight shaking with pain. You would be crazy to do this shoot! Please let them know that you won't make it.' Looking back, it seems so silly, but my attitude was to continue living my life as normal. The only way I could cope was by compartmentalising my feelings and moving on.

I did manage to see sense and cancel the photo shoot, and I was relieved to rest and recuperate for the next few days, making sure to add an iron supplement into my daily routine to help boost my energy levels. On 10 March, I left Sophia at home with Wes for a couple of hours while I popped out to a recording studio in Bray, Co. Wicklow, to talk about my fertility journey on the *Everymum* podcast. For the first time that year, there were no hugs or handshakes, just a polite wave over the mics and a reminder to sanitise my hands. Covid had arrived.

From that point on, life as we knew it changed dramatically. The then-Taoiseach, Leo Varadkar, made his impactful speech on 12 March 2020 in Washington DC (where he was staying ahead of what ought to have been St Patrick's

Day parades) and the country shut down. It was a frightening time, with people falling ill or losing their jobs and businesses closing, but it also marked a further shift in my lifestyle. When that first lockdown was announced, I experienced an almost physical sensation of relief. Of course, we watched in shock as the news reported chaos and horrifying loss of life in Northern Italy and China. It was a frightening time because so much about this illness was unknown, but there was a strange paradox between the mayhem unfolding in the outside world and feeling safe and secure in our little bubble at home. For the first time since Sophia was born, there was no pressure for me to be anywhere. While my schedule had certainly changed pace when she arrived, it still felt like a constant juggle between my professional obligations and motherhood, although the latter mattered far more to me. Now I didn't have to think about tomorrow's work commitments and how I might manage it all. Up until this point, I had pushed myself to return to some element of normal work life: my logic was that because I didn't give birth to Sophia, I didn't really deserve to take time off. I can be pretty hard on myself sometimes. I was lucky to have Mum and Wes to help out, but even so, I was finding it difficult to establish a balance. Most new parents experience similar challenges and compromises have to be made.

I could work from home quite easily; however, it was a stressful time for Wes. He had to close the business immediately and make sure over 125 staff, many of whom had been working for the family for years, were looked after and that they could reopen safely when government restrictions allowed. He spent a lot of time on the phone, and because life felt unpredictable, he worried a lot. We also missed seeing our families, especially with a newborn at home. Mum and Dad didn't see Sophia again until the summer, when she was six months old. Mum in particular found that very hard, and she FaceTimed Sophia every day so that she wouldn't forget her voice and face.

For me, home was an oasis of calm and contentment compared to the turbulence across the world, and with so much widespread suffering and anxiety, we felt extremely grateful to have each other. I could feel myself unwinding with each day that passed, savouring the family time together. I'd established a little routine to help bring some normality into our daily lives. Every morning, I'd get some housework done, play with Sophia, do a home workout while she was having her midday nap, cook a meal for us and enjoy the sunny weather outside in the garden. I had told my family and a couple of close friends about the miscarriage, but otherwise I'd managed to move on from it, and our surrogacy plans for July were still in place.

By the second week of April, I recall feeling unusually tired. It would get to 2.30 or 3 p.m. and a power nap would seem appealing. I was keeping up my daily home Pilates and weight-training workouts at the time, and I remember thinking I'd better get them done in the mornings because

I didn't have the energy for them after lunch. I couldn't put my finger on it, I just felt different. In fact, one afternoon in mid-April after I'd given Sophia her bottle, I nodded off with her on the sofa and Wes cheekily captured it on camera. Now, of course, it all makes sense.

The week of my birthday arrived and the tiredness continued, but I perked up when Wes suggested we have a barbecue outside to celebrate because it was a beautiful bright, sunny day. I walked into our kitchen on the morning of my birthday and found the whole room colourfully decorated with balloons, banners and confetti. He had got up early and made the room look festive because he felt bad that I was at home in lockdown. He'd bought a chocolate fudge cake for me and we toasted the occasion with a glass of bubbly with our breakfast before going out for a walk in the local park with Sophia. We ended the evening with a family Zoom quiz – while it was still a novelty! It was a lovely, relaxed day, followed by an early night because Sophia was still waking for a 3 a.m. feed.

When I woke up the following day, 18 April, I remember feeling strangely sad and emotional. We'd finished the bottle of champagne during my birthday barbecue the day before and enjoyed a gin and tonic in the evening once Sophia was asleep, but we didn't go overboard. Yet I couldn't stop sobbing. Wes came into the kitchen at one point and said, 'Rosie, what is wrong with you? Are you OK? I've caught you crying about five times today.' I'd cry at a dog video on Facebook, a sad advert on the TV or from the sudden wave of nostalgia you get from looking through old family photos. I went to bed early again that night feeling tired and lightheaded, and the next morning the feeling still lingered. I wasn't used to feeling dizzy, so after my shower, I thought, Maybe I'll take a pregnancy test, just in case. I always seem to have tests in my bathroom cupboard – I must have spent a fortune on them at this stage. I used to buy them in different chemist's because I'd feel too embarrassed to keep going into the one pharmacy asking for yet another test.

I had no idea what stage I was at in my cycle because I hadn't had a period since the miscarriage, but when I took the test, two very strong pink lines swiftly appeared. I tried to do the calculations in my head and worked out that I must be around six-and-a-half weeks pregnant at that stage. I stared at the test for a couple of minutes before popping it in my pocket and wandering downstairs to the kitchen, where Wes was playing with Sophia. 'Oh, look, this just happened,' I said, ever-so-casually showing it to him.

We looked at each other and he carefully said, 'OK.' I could see that we were both thinking exactly the same thing: that we couldn't face going through another one of those distressing, exhausting miscarriages. I didn't feel particularly excited about it – in fact, my first glum thoughts were, Oh no, this again. I left it for a day or two to see if there would be any initial signs of the pregnancy failing, as they usually did at about that point. Early the following week, when nothing had happened, I decided to send a text to the consultant obstetrician and gynaecologist I'd previously seen to get some advice, and I explained to him that I'd had a painful miscarriage the previous month. 'Come into me this week if you can and we'll check you out,' he replied. So that's what I did, assuming that I was around seven weeks pregnant by then.

When he scanned me, he was able to find a sac but no embryo. The doctor said, 'Well, there's a gestational sac and I can see that it has implanted in a very good position in the fundus of the uterus, but it appears to be empty, and if you are seven weeks pregnant, we should be able to detect a foetus and a heartbeat at this point.' My heart sank a little bit. When I'd seen the sac, my hopes had risen, but as the doctor explained to me about anembryonic pregnancies, where a gestational sac develops in the uterus but an embryo doesn't form, I could feel the disappointment take hold.

'Will you be OK?' he asked, as we discussed what this might mean.

'Yes, I'm fine. I've been through so much – it really doesn't affect me as intensely any more because I have a beautiful baby to go home to. I'll be OK.' Even though I was putting on a brave face while feeling sad, I knew that I would recover. I always did.

The doctor said, 'Look, it does happen that a woman gets her dates wrong, for whatever reason, so come back to me next week and we'll check you again. Then we can discuss our options.'

I rang Wes on the way home to tell him the news that I was pregnant but that it was an empty sac and it looked like it would end at some stage soon. He was as sympathetic and supportive as ever, but I knew that this would be tough on him as well. I went home and mentally prepared myself for another miscarriage, convinced that any change in my early pregnancy symptoms meant that the pregnancy was ending. How would I face going into Holles Street for another scan after a pregnancy loss, I wondered over that weekend. However, when I woke up on Monday, I still felt nauseated and exhausted. For the first time, I wondered had I actually got my dates wrong. Maybe I wasn't as far along as I'd thought. After all the upset of the miscarriage the previous month, my system was a little unsettled, so my calculations might have been off. I could feel the first flickers of excitement and hope beginning.

Three days later, I went back for a scan. The doctor peered at the screen and so did I, checking the sac carefully. Then I thought I spotted something. 'What's that?' I said, pointing at the screen.

'That is an embryo with a beating heart.'

I burst into tears in front of the doctor and the nurse who was in the room with us. 'Oh my gosh, I've never got to the point of seeing a heartbeat before!' I couldn't believe it. I'd been ready to tell him that I was preparing for a natural miscarriage, and instead, we were looking at a beating heart and a tiny developing baby. I was totally overwhelmed at the news. The doctor told me that I was probably just over six weeks pregnant – so I *had* got my dates wrong – and reassured me that everything looked normal.

As soon as I left the hospital I rang Wes. 'You'll never believe this, they've detected an embryo with a beating heart!'

There was a long pause and then he said, 'What? That's crazy!' We allowed ourselves the tiniest bit of excitement, then agreed that we'd take each step as it came and, for the time being, we'd keep the news to ourselves. It was hard, because I'd always shared it with my family, but after the previous miscarriage, I knew that I couldn't put them through that again. It was too much.

As the week continued, my morning nausea increased, and I remember looking at my lower tummy and thinking that I looked very bloated for someone not yet seven weeks pregnant. Even at that early stage, I had been prescribed daily progesterone, baby aspirin and heparin injections to support the new pregnancy, and I assumed that my body must have been responding to the medication by retaining water. Luckily, I was going back to the doctor the following week for a further scan, so I could ask him plenty of questions. I spent the next few days doing my best to distract myself by reading, listening to interesting science podcasts and spending plenty of time in the garden with Sophia. She has always been fascinated by trees, flowers and birds, and we love the magic of experiencing the natural world around us through her eyes.

May 7 arrived and I woke early to drive to the National Maternity Hospital in Holles Street for my third scan in as many weeks. The streets were deserted in the height of the first lockdown, and it felt strange to be venturing out of the safety of my home. I was stopped at a Garda checkpoint on the way into the city centre, and they ushered me through when I told them that I was on my way for an early pregnancy scan. Even saying the words out loud filled me with a tingle of excitement. I couldn't wait to see how my little embryo was doing.

At the hospital, while I rolled my top up over my stomach and settled myself on the bed, my consultant – Master of the National Maternity Hospital, Professor Shane Higgins – and I chatted about the lovely weather and the strangeness of Covid as he squirted on the ultrasound gel. There was a silence while he swished the transducer over my tummy. 'Oh,' he said.

I had already spotted the baby with its tiny pulsing heartbeat, but there was another strange shape to the left of it. 'There are two, aren't there?' I said, shrieking.

'Just let me check,' he calmly replied, peering closely at the image. Up on the screen, we could see the embryo that we'd examined in such detail the first time, and then he moved the wand across and there it was, another baby. 'Yes, it's twins,' the doctor said.

'Holy shit!' That was all I could think of to say! 'Oh, my gosh, I can't believe there's more than one in there.' Now it all made sense, those feelings of nausea and dizziness. Double the hormones! I lay there in shock as the doctor and nurse conferred to see whether the twins were identical or fraternal. 'Well, I can see two separate membranes,' Professor Higgins said, inspecting the pair of tiny curled-up shapes. 'Hmm, I think they're monochorionic diamniotic,' and he went on to explain that each twin had a separate amniotic sac, but they shared a placenta.

'If I'm having twins, does that mean my fertilised egg split in two?'

'Yes, exactly,' he said, explaining that with fraternal twins there would be two separate eggs, each fertilised, but here, one egg had divided and the result was identical twins. They could tell all of this at seven weeks, I thought. How amazing.

I rushed out to the car, my mind racing, hands trembling as I fumbled around in my bag for the keys. I just couldn't process this information quickly enough. As soon as I got into the car, for the third week in a row following a scan, I rang Wes. 'You'll never guess what. It's twins! There are two in there, both with heartbeats.' Poor Wes, he just couldn't think what to say. After so many disappointments and dashed hopes, he never imagined he'd get a call like this. But we decided to be sensible and not get our hopes up too much at such an early, vulnerable stage of the pregnancy, so we agreed to wait another few weeks before telling anyone – apart from Mum and Dad, of course. I couldn't keep this news from them.

When I rang my parents a short while later, asking Mum to put me on speakerphone, I said, 'I hope you're sitting down. I have some pretty incredible news.'

They both let out a shriek in shock and amazement as I revealed that I had discovered I was pregnant just after my birthday and my consultant had detected a beating heart at the previous week's scan. 'But that's not all! There are two in there. Twins!' Of course, they were ecstatic, but cautious. I could tell how excited my mum was, but she reminded me that it was still early days and not to raise my hopes too much. Apart from Mum and Dad, we didn't tell anybody, not even Wes's parents, because it still felt too uncertain.

For the next few weeks, I went in for scans once a week and the growth and development of my two little babies looked increasingly reassuring. More to the point, I was experiencing all the symptoms of first-trimester pregnancy. I was constantly exhausted with the kind of heavy, eye-watering tiredness I used to associate with jet lag, and I needed to take a nap every afternoon. I used to snuggle up in bed beside Sophia's cot when she had her afternoon snoozes. And I was constantly ravenous. My body was building a complex support system for two babies, so I couldn't get enough food. I craved bland carbohydrates the most and would often wake during the night feeling very hungry and have to go downstairs to make a big bowl of porridge. I can still remember making a huge pasta bake with roast veggies and vegan mozzarella at around eight or nine weeks pregnant and Wes's jaw dropped. 'You'll never eat all that – it's enough for a family of six.' It took me two days!

It was strange to want to eat everything while feeling nauseated at the same time, but it was the kind of nausea that felt worse with an empty stomach. Pregnancy hormones are well-known for heightening your sense of smell and, coupled with nausea, it can make even the most inoffensive objects smell horrendous. Sophia's bottle steriliser made me feel sick, the woody smell of the inside of the drawer in our coffee table was bizarrely unpleasant, and one day in May, Wes decided to fry scallops and I had to leave the kitchen for hours. I also went off green veggies, which was particularly strange for me. I normally eat a lot of greens to support my iron and calcium intake, but I couldn't stomach them for much of the pregnancy. Sulphur-rich brassica vegetables, like broccoli, kale and cabbage, were especially unappetising, yet I went through a phase of really enjoying sliced vine tomatoes sprinkled with sea salt and black pepper. The most unusual aversion was tea. I usually love coffee in the morning and tea in the afternoon and evening, but even the thought of a simple cup almost made me retch. I couldn't bear to see the box of teabags in our cupboard, yet I still looked forward to my morning coffee, despite switching to decaffeinated. Muesli was another odd one – I think it was mainly the raisins scattered innocently throughout it. I found that smelling fresh lemons and citrus oil really helped and I kept a diffuser for essential oils in the kitchen, as well as bland crackers beside the bed. I drank a lot of fresh ginger tea too, although I didn't think it made much of a difference to the feelings of nausea.

The cravings were weird and wonderful too and they seemed to change by the day. I often wondered if they were all in my head, but the desire for certain tastes and textures was so physically intense that I could barely think about anything else. Sometimes salty foods like popcorn, olives and salted nuts hit the spot, while stodgy foods featured heavily too. Toast, noodles, noodles on toast! Throughout the entire pregnancy I craved and ate a lot of fruit, especially grapes, pineapple, mango and watermelon. I often wondered if my body was telling me that it required certain essential nutrients. Perhaps it needed extra vitamin C to support absorption of the iron required to help build enough blood for a twin pregnancy. I used to buy grapes and berries and pop them into the freezer, to enjoy them icy cold with a cup of ginger and lemon tea. Wes often had to head out to the local shop to satisfy my sudden, random cravings and he mostly did so uncomplainingly. I remember a night in week nine where I was craving white flour so strongly that I couldn't go to bed without making scones. I stayed up late baking them, and as soon as I bit into the first one, I thought, *Ahh, that hit the spot.*

I had scans fortnightly throughout the second trimester. They were so frequent because a twin pregnancy with one placenta is considered high-risk. My scans at eight, nine and ten weeks showed a normal growth trajectory for both babies and healthy foetal heart rates. Everything looked very positive, and the speed of their development amazed me. By nine weeks, we could see their first tiny, jerky movements as they began to look more and more like little humans. Professor Higgins was confident enough to say that we could tell more family and friends at ten weeks, because he could see no reason why it wouldn't be a healthy pregnancy. Feeling horribly nauseated every day, as much as I didn't enjoy it, was also very reassuring. There was a couple of days where I didn't feel sick and I remember saying to Mum, 'I'm awfully worried that something is wrong,' and then the nausea came back again. It's not enjoyable but I still found it encouraging.

We had a scare one night when I was ten-and-a-half weeks pregnant. Wes and I were sitting on the sofa in our sitting room watching TV before bed. I was snuggled up in my pyjamas under a blanket, and as I stood up to let the dogs out before heading upstairs, I felt a sudden spurt of warm fluid from underneath me. I whipped around in horror to see a puddle of blood on the sofa, and as I quickly looked over at Wes, I saw his jaw dropping in shock. I stared down at my blood-soaked pyjamas, heart sinking. *This is the gestational point at which I lost the pregnancy in March – it's going to happen again.* My mind was racing; how could this happen to us after what we'd been through? I dreaded the idea of a miscarriage at this stage. I couldn't take the pain again, I thought, as we cleaned up the blood. It was approaching midnight and, not wanting to disturb Professor Higgins that late, I sadly trudged upstairs to shower and change, dreading what the next few hours might hold.

When I stepped out of the shower and plucked up the courage to check again, the bleeding had strangely stopped and I didn't have any cramping either. I had no idea what was going on in my body. I slipped into bed but couldn't really sleep, tossing and turning for the rest of the night, my mind racing with possible scenarios. I woke early, feeling my anxiety levels rising. At 7 a.m. I sent a text to Professor Higgins, who suggested I go straight in to the emergency department in Holles Street. However, as I was driving in, something about this incident felt different. I could still feel the hormones surging through my system, unlike with previous miscarriages where they'd disappeared a few days beforehand. The familiar nausea and tiredness were still there.

The staff in the emergency department were very sweet and supportive, arranging for me to have a scan immediately. I held my breath as the cool ultrasound gel was spread across my lower tummy and, there on the screen, I watched my two healthy babies dancing around inside me. I could see them doing little twirls and somersaults and their legs had grown a bit longer since the previous scan. I cried with relief. The timing had made me think that the same thing was happening all over again, but I could see now that it wasn't. I whispered a thank you to the nurse and asked what could possibly have happened. 'There's so much blood flow in your abdominal area that it could have been a little growth spurt in your uterus that caused the bleeding.' There was no evidence of it being any kind of blood clot or other issue, but because I was injecting a blood thinner daily, it probably appeared worse than it was.

The lovely nurse who was looking after me had identical twins, and she told me that it could also be that the uterus grows faster with twins to make space for their growth, so there might be bleeding as a result. 'Have you been feeling period pains?' she said.

'Yes, I've had cramps in the last week.'

'Well, that's down to your uterus stretching,' she reassured me. 'There doesn't seem to be anything else wrong.'

As soon as I could, I rang Wes with the good news that it was just a scare, and we both breathed a sigh of relief. I can remember the initial sense of horror and fear as the bleeding started, and wondering how I could get through it again – but, thankfully, I didn't need to. It was all going to be OK. It really seemed like a miracle.

That first trimester seemed to drag on for ever. The days passed very slowly and I was aware of what stage I was at all the time. I'd methodically count off the days: 'eight weeks and five days', 'eight weeks and six days', 'ten weeks and four days' and so on. Time seemed to stretch into eternity while we waited for that twelve-week mark. Every test and scan was a milestone, bringing us another bit closer to safety.

Just before eleven weeks, we decided to have a screening test called the Harmony test, which is a blood test designed to analyse cell-free DNA in maternal blood to check for genetic issues such as Down syndrome (trisomy 21), Edwards' syndrome (trisomy 18) or Patau syndrome (trisomy 13). Not every expectant mother has it, but I requested it because I was aware that, as I was over the age of thirty-five, I would be at higher risk for certain issues, so I wanted the peace of mind.

One other wonderful thing about the test is that it reveals the gender of the baby or babies, if you want to find out. I'm not one of these people who has the patience to wait for such a big surprise, so I was desperate to know and to share the news with my family. I'd wanted to know for Sophia as well because it gave me something to look forward to and plan for – and we could start thinking about baby names, which I've always enjoyed.

I got the test result back within a week. A nurse rang from the clinic and her first words were, 'I've got good news for you.' I breathed an enormous sigh of relief. Your mind can go to some pretty strange places when you're waiting for the result of a test like that, and I'd been so anxious that there would be something wrong that their gender wasn't a priority. So, when the nurse said, 'Good news, we didn't detect any chromosomal abnormalities with them,' I had to sit down for a second. 'Thank you so much,' I managed. 'That's just the best news.'

'I believe you also asked to find out their gender?'

'Oh yes,' I said. I'd almost forgotten in my relief.

'Well, I'm delighted to tell you that you're expecting two boys!'

Two boys. Oh, my goodness, I thought. I'd have been thrilled to be having either, but two boys would make Wes the happiest man in the world. He adores his little girl, and all he wanted then was healthy twins, but I knew that, deep down, he'd always wanted a son. Now, he was going to have two. I knew that he'd be absolutely delighted.

But I had planned to keep it a secret from him for another couple of days. It was Monday 8 June, and in two days I'd be twelve weeks pregnant. It was finally time to tell the rest of my family, with the extra bonus of revealing the gender. For the next couple of days I was like a child excitedly waiting for Christmas. I organised a Zoom meeting for the whole family, ignoring any excuses. We were well and truly over Zoom at that point, but I insisted that we have a chat at 5 p.m. on Wednesday evening. One of my brothers revealed to my mum that he was worried that something was wrong. 'Why does she need to chat to us?' Mum said vaguely, 'Oh, I don't know. She misses everyone, I suppose.' I found it harder to keep the secret from Wes, though. I'm the worst liar and he knows me very well. He spent the next couple of days trying to get it out of me and I eventually said, 'Look you're going to have to stop because I won't be able to keep it a secret, so if you want a surprise on Wednesday, don't press me any further.'

Meanwhile, I put my gender-reveal plans into action. I bought a chocolate cake, carefully cut a hole in the centre and scooped out the filling. I poured blue sprinkles into the hole and covered it up again with cake. As I popped two candles on top, one pink and one blue, I reflected that it had only been twelve months since I'd done the same for Sophia. We'd found out her gender on 11 June 2019. What a year it had been.

We all gathered on the Zoom call, with Wes, Sophia and me sitting around the kitchen table beside my parents in their house, the cake in front of us, and my two brothers with their partners in their homes in London. After a few minutes of general chat, I spoke up. 'Well, we've got you on this call because we have some news to share,' I said. I could see their ears pricking up, wondering if there was going to be some juicy gossip. I continued. 'The news is that we're going to be expanding our family this November.'

Everyone's face dropped. I could see my brother Hubie counting on his fingers to work out what month it had all happened! 'That's wonderful,' he said. 'We know you guys wanted to go down the surrogacy route again and I'm so pleased that it's worked.'

I couldn't help but smile at the misunderstanding. I gave them a second, then said, 'But the really exciting news is that I'm the one who's pregnant!' My twelve-week bump was tiny, but I pulled up my top proudly and showed them my gently rounded tummy. I gave them a minute to process this, then I said, 'Actually, that's not all. There's more news to come. We're having identical twins. There are two babies in there!' I could see the shock on everyone's faces, before they erupted in excitement. I was asked about identical twins and how on earth it had all happened.

'So, this is all natural?' one of my brothers said.

'Yes,' I said. 'All absolutely natural. We weren't planning any of this!'

Then after the initial shock of it had settled a little, I prepared for the final act. 'And now, we're going to find out the gender!' I was the only person who knew at this point, so the excitement levels were high. Mum and Dad were squealing with anticipation, and Wes was assuring everyone that he really didn't have any idea. I pulled over the cake, lit the two candles and we blew them out. Then, using my mum's serrated cake knife, Wes and I cut into it and out tumbled a cascade of blue sprinkles. Wes yelped, 'Oh my goodness, we're having boys!'

What a lockdown surprise! It meant so much to me to share this lovely and unexpected news with the family. They'd been with me right from the start of my journey, and telling them made it all seem more real. It was finally happening, after everything we'd been through. We recorded the chat and I've looked back at it many times since, enjoying the looks of surprise and excitement on everyone's faces. It felt like such a special milestone to be able to announce this double miracle pregnancy. I also loved not having to hide the news from them any more. Later that week, we did the same thing with Wes's family, before telling three close friends and delivering the news in exactly the same way as we had on the first call. We didn't have cake every time – but I took such pride in showing off my bump and revealing the gender of our surprise babies.

Our surrogate had been on my mind throughout my first trimester, because she had been planning the second half of her year around potentially being pregnant with our child. I felt a little nervous to tell her the news that I had naturally conceived twins, but she was kind, gracious and incredibly happy for us when later that week, I sent her a message in Ukrainian using a translator app. She said it was the most wonderful news that Sophia would have two siblings so close in age and she wished me the best for my pregnancy. I thanked her again for all that she had done for us, and it felt strange to tell her that we wouldn't need her help again after all.

I did ask Professor Higgins how he thought it had happened for us after so many losses and he admitted that he wasn't sure. 'There's really no scientific or medical explanation I can give you, but in my experience, it often happens when people have stopped trying.' He gave the example of couples who would conceive naturally after having IVF treatment or going through the surrogacy process, as we did. I explained that we'd stopped thinking about it and stopped trying and that the text message from our surrogate at the beginning of the year had been a huge source of relief. I felt that our more relaxed lifestyle in lockdown probably had something to do with it too. Despite huge advancements in medical science, elements of nature and the human body remain a mystery. I do know that my whole pace of life changed in 2020 and I would love for it to stay like that. Being in lockdown taught me to live in a much more simple, mindful way and to appreciate the small moments. And I was able to drink my first cup of tea by week sixteen. Things were definitely looking up.

CHAPTER 9

A SURPRISE ENDING

Telling my family and close friends that I was pregnant was a huge relief. It felt so good to share the news and not have to carry the burden of a secret around any longer. It felt even better to be able to share a happy story with them after all the struggles of the previous few years. They'd been with me on the rollercoaster, sharing the ups and downs of our journey, and now we'd given them something to really celebrate and look forward to.

Privately, I was experiencing a range of different emotions and some were unexpected. It was primarily joy and elation but also a huge amount of shock and surprise. I was also battling feelings of guilt because I had tried to be a voice of reassurance for women and couples dealing with infertility since announcing that Sophia was *in utero* through gestational surrogacy, and now I was in a very different space. I'd grown comfortable in my role of someone who'd been through it and who could be a supportive presence, spreading the message that fertility problems are more common than you'd imagine and should be normalised to help those suffering alone to feel listened to and understood. I got a lot of emails, from women in particular, who told me about their battles to conceive and their struggles with miscarriages, IVF or surrogacy, and I was only too pleased to support them by sharing my own difficulties. I felt that, at the very least, I could use my own experiences to help others.

Now, I'd suddenly become pregnant with two healthy babies and initially I found it difficult to reconcile my feelings. I feel such compassion and empathy for anyone going through what we experienced, but the guilt I felt was unanticipated, and I suppose it put me off sharing our news with anyone outside the family for a long time. It felt like survivor's guilt, in a way – a feeling that I shouldn't be this lucky. I was also faced with having to redefine my sense of self. I'd become comfortable with the idea that I was the girl who couldn't have a baby, that my body wasn't functioning in the way it was designed to. It had become part of the conversation in my head about myself and tied into how I viewed myself; I could be proud of lots of other parts of my life, but pregnancy was just something that hadn't worked out for me. Now, I had to go through the process of reversing all I thought I knew about myself. It felt strange and unfamiliar for a long time.

Wes had to go through a sense of redefining who he was as well, from accepting that we might be childless to becoming a father of three in the space of just a year. It had been our dream to have three or even four children (now, maybe three is enough!) but we'd made peace with the idea that it may not come true. So, for most of the pregnancy, Wes would stare at my growing bump and exclaim, 'I can't believe you're pregnant. I never thought I would see the day!' We talked about the huge changes in our lives and I had to face up to all of my feelings towards it, good and bad. I made a significant effort not to bottle up my thoughts and to share what was going on for me with him. As I have said before, my advice to anyone going through struggles with infertility is to talk about it with family and close friends because sharing these sometimes huge, frightening emotions is one of the most healing steps you can take. It certainly made a big difference to the healing process for us.

In this, I found Mum a huge help. She's the kind of person everyone goes to for advice. She likes to talk through things and consider why you're feeling a certain way. We've been brought up to be open about our problems and concerns. So, if I called her and said, 'I'm feeling really down today and feeling guilty,' she wouldn't dismiss it or tell me that I'd feel better before long – instead, she'd talk me through it, and I learned how to handle my emotions in a healthy way.

I owe both my parents such a lot. It's important to me to live my life honestly, to embrace every aspect of who I am and not to hide any part of it. We're all just humans trying to navigate our way through life, adapting as we go, living shared experiences and facing uncertainty about the future.

However, it had taken me a long time to say anything publicly about our fertility struggles because I didn't feel that I'd dealt with it fully myself. I prefer not to put my experiences and their associated emotions into words until I've categorised them in my head, worked out what they mean for me and why I'm feeling them. I wasn't consciously hiding our baby situation from friends and extended family, but we just weren't ready to tell them until we announced publicly that Sophia was on her way in 2019.

We chose to make our announcement on Instagram because I could spend time thinking about what I wanted to say and composing a post that would be honest and heartfelt and that would express the right message. I wanted to share that we were going through the surrogacy process for valid medical reasons and to give as much detail as I could in one caption about why we'd made our choices. Instagram was the most controlled way that we could release the information because, as I've learned, every news item that comes from an initial post is more or less copied from the caption, so all the information is there should anyone want it.

We waited until the exact same week in 2020 to announce my pregnancy with the twins. I knew instinctively when

I'd be ready to share our news – when I'd worked through all of the unexpected emotions I'd had and felt comfortable with this huge change in my life. I remember meeting friends for brunch in early July, when the country opened up again between lockdowns, and feeling that I needed to disguise my pregnancy. By sixteen weeks, with twins, I was definitely showing, but I arrived at the restaurant wearing an oversized blazer and a big scarf – despite the warm July weather. I didn't feel ready to tell them because we were in a public place, and I didn't want people overhearing any fuss being made. However, by eighteen weeks, I was at the halfway point of the pregnancy and felt ready to tell friends and then the wider world. We asked Wes's mum to take a photo of us and Sophia to post online with our pregnancy-announcement caption. I wore a white dress to show my baby bump, which I thought was enormous at the time but was actually quite neat. By the time November came around, I would know all about huge bumps! This is what we said:

> We have some news! @wesquirke and I are beyond overjoyed to announce that we're expecting identical twin boys this November. We're absolutely thrilled to complete our family and for our daughter Sophia to have two siblings so close in age to her.
>
> As I've spoken openly about this year, we struggled with fourteen pregnancy losses over the past few years and a challenging fertility journey before finally welcoming Sophia last November by gestational surrogate. I

was told that I would probably never be able to carry my own baby due to a suspected immune system dysfunction, which numerous different medical treatments failed to rectify. So for this to just happen naturally, and to have twins too by complete chance, is an absolute dream come true for us. My doctor can't offer a medical explanation for why I have been able to sustain this pregnancy and it will probably always remain one of life's mysteries. However, we found out I was pregnant after the first month of lockdown when I was far more physically relaxed than I've been in years and enjoying the slow pace of family life at home, despite the anxiety and sadness in the outside world. So perhaps that time out from the stress of busy everyday life made all the difference. We still can't quite believe it ourselves and it's taken a long time to properly process it and feel ready to share the news. As if 2020 hasn't already been packed with enough surprises! Fertility miracles may take some time, but they really can happen in the most unexpected and magical ways. As always, sending so much love to those of you still on your baby journey. Never give up hope

#twinpregnancy #novemberbabies #month5 #halfway-there #fertilityawareness

I was determined that the announcement would be positive and honest, as I'm conscious of all the people out there who are enduring such heartbreak while I have been unbelievably lucky. So, this was very much the way we approached it. And when we did announce our pregnancy, the love and support we received was overwhelming. It was beyond what we could have expected. I was actually moved to tears by it. When Wes and I were dealing with pregnancy losses, I used to find friends' pregnancy announcements difficult to see, to be honest. I'd feel huge joy and happiness for them but still a lot of sadness for myself. Following our big announcement, we received an outpouring of love and support that was extremely uplifting. Having said all of that, I was so aware of the people out there who would have loved to be in my situation and who weren't or couldn't be, so I wanted to be as sensitive as possible. I've struggled a lot over the years with feeling responsible for the way other people feel, but I realise now that I can't be. I can only be responsible for my own actions and emotions and how I react to things. Thus, after this huge outpouring of love and support, I gave myself permission to be excited, to look forward to November when the boys would arrive and to give thanks for my good fortune. I find that others appreciate when you share your vulnerabilities and challenges because nobody has a perfect life, but everyone enjoys a happy outcome.

I remember arriving at fourteen weeks pregnant so clearly because the nausea and tiredness lifted almost overnight and I started feeling much more energetic. I was safely into the next trimester, which felt incredibly exciting. After so many disappointments, it was strange and unfamiliar to have reached that far. But now that I had, I was determined to enjoy my pregnancy as much as I could, which included taking regular exercise and eating well. Under the encouragement and advice of Professor Higgins, I continued to go to the gym three times a week for prenatal training with my trainer, Jessica Kavanagh. She split the thirty-minute sessions into two lower-body and one upper-body per week, and they included a range of safe exercises to encourage blood flow and lymphatic drainage and support and strengthen my shoulders, legs, back muscles and pelvic area to carry two growing babies. They were very much tailored to my own abilities and built around my pre-pregnancy regime because Jessi has been training me since 2017. It was also important for my mental health and clarity to continue to work out, and I believe it made a big difference to my postnatal recovery. I've been practising Pilates since the age of eighteen, and before Sophia was born I went to classes at Pilates Plus Dublin three or four times a week, so I'm familiar with the exercises I need to do to build and maintain my core muscles safely. I knew that awareness would help after pregnancy too. I'm lucky to have a knowledgeable and very well qualified personal trainer, but any good trainer should have experience of prenatal training and talk to their client about any potential or existing medical issues, like high blood pressure, low iron or previous injuries, and will recommend exercises that work for pregnancy. From weeks sixteen to twenty-six, I swam two or three times a week and found it helped to rectify lingering stiffness in my lower back and pelvis. I also did my Kegel, or pelvic-floor, exercises, which any pregnant woman knows are essential – I tried to remember to do them when driving.

I've been eating a plant-based diet for a decade and continued to do so throughout my pregnancy. When the nausea and cravings of the first trimester lifted, I was able to focus on eating sources of complete protein, complex carbs, healthy fats and lots of colourful fruit and vegetables. A typical day featured three meals and a couple of snacks, with a bowl of porridge for breakfast topped with seeds, chopped nuts and berries, followed by lentil soup and a salad for lunch or a homemade chickpea, avocado and carrot salad, with a bean stew, a veggie burger or a tofu-and-vegetable stir-fry for dinner. I snacked on fruit, vegan protein bars and protein shakes or I'd mix protein powder into soya or coconut yoghurt. My carb mania settled down in the second trimester, and I didn't have any significant cravings, apart from fruit, so I munched on berries, grapes, watermelon, pineapples and apples. But by the time I got to week twenty-nine or thirty, I started to crave stodgier carbohydrates again, so I added more sweet potato and butternut squash, brown bread, wholegrain rice and pasta to my diet. I felt like my body was telling me it was time to fatten up these babies.

As you probably know, folic acid is crucial in the first trimester of pregnancy to help prevent neural tube defects, such as spina bifida, and I was careful to ensure I was also consuming enough iron, calcium and magnesium to support a twin pregnancy. The latter two minerals also helped to reduce cramps in my legs. I designed my own diet and supplement plan based on the nutrient requirements for a twin pregnancy, with vitamins D3, B12 and DHA a focus too. I took a good-quality daily pregnancy supplement and made sure that my diet was well-balanced and packed with fibre-rich whole plant foods.

When I was about twenty-three weeks pregnant, we went on a little summer break to our family holiday home in Wexford, taking Sophia to the beach and enjoying strolls through the fields. After quite a long walk on the beach, I was ravenous. When we found the local shop, I spotted a shelf of Pot Noodle and I thought, bingo! Wes nearly fell over in shock when we got home and I boiled the kettle to soak them, before hungrily digging in. They were hot, spicy and delicious, just what I needed. All the way through my pregnancy, I'd been careful to eat well, avoid processed foods and ensure I was providing the babies with all the nutrition they required and keeping my energy levels up. I find that your body tells you what it needs – and right then, it needed curry Pot Noodles!

Of course, at the same time as being overjoyed, I was naturally a bit anxious about the pregnancy. I seemed to give myself something to worry about every week. I felt very well throughout the second and third trimesters and the scans were so positive that it seemed almost too good to be true. After all we'd been through, it felt like a complete miracle. And I didn't have any of the issues that can arise in a twin pregnancy either. There is a condition called twin-to-twin transfusion syndrome (TTTS) in pregnancies where there is a shared placenta, as mine was. This can lead to one twin receiving more blood and nutrients and growing bigger than the other, but the fortnightly scans with a twin special-ist showed that there was no indication of this happening. Both boys were developing normally and displayed similar growth trajectories. As the weeks passed and I reached the initial stage of viability at twenty-four weeks, then got to twenty-six weeks, I gradually began to relax. I understood that if the worst happened and I was to deliver them early, paediatric medicine is now so advanced that the twins would have a good chance of survival. Each subsequent block of two weeks was a milestone on the journey, each scan reas-suring me that everything was going well, and I finally began to slowly trust that it would all work out.

Even though I was carrying twins, with all of the potential risks that go with that, Wes and I were a lot more relaxed about the prospect of becoming parents than we'd been with Sophia. Before she came along, we didn't know how to change a nappy or make a bottle, but we'd learned so much in the previous year about looking after newborns that the idea of two more didn't faze us at all. With the first baby, I think you go into overdrive. I was a baby marketer's dream, buying every gadget and gizmo I thought might make all of our lives easier. I used to check Sophia's breathing all the time, especially when she was a tiny newborn, and for the first twelve weeks I went through night terrors, where

I'd dream that I was lying on her or that I had fallen asleep with her and smothered her during the night. I'd wake up cradling the pillow, thinking it was Sophia, before realising that she was fast asleep in her cot beside the bed. It happened to Wes as well, and we both thought we were going mad in the beginning. But now we know that it's all part of having a newborn and the joy and worries that come with it. I used to spend a lot of time wondering how I would be able to look after this little person for the next eighteen years, overwhelmed by the responsibility of it all. I'm sure many new parents feel that way.

I was surprised to find that, despite my pregnancy worries, I was still less anxious about expecting the twins than I was with Sophia, whereas I'd been anticipating it to be the other way around. I thought the very idea of having twins would send me into anxiety overdrive, but I felt as if I was more in control with this pregnancy: I was the one carrying them, nourishing them and looking after them. With Sophia, I wasn't in control of anything. Of course, we were sent regular updates and all the medical information we needed, but we were thousands of miles away from Sophia, in a different country, entrusting our hopes and dreams to a stranger. We'd pore over her scan pictures and videos, but this time, I was the one going to the scans. It felt much more reassuring to be the one in control of everything, except of course the birth itself, which was to be a scheduled C-section at thirty-six weeks. Friends had assured me that the procedure would be painless and that I'd just feel a lot of tugging. The idea of having a caesarean delivery didn't worry me – I was happy to follow my consultant's advice. And I'd have Wes by my side, feeling confident because he'd watched so many episodes of *One Born Every Minute*! He'd recorded a special episode of the programme on twins and I wondered if he was preparing himself or me.

Between weeks twenty-eight and thirty-five, I had to really slow down and spend most of the day on my backside resting because the combined weight of the twins was very heavy. I was swollen, aching and had to be heaved up off the sofa by Wes every night. I made grunting sounds as I hoisted myself out of bed in the morning, and the soles of my feet ached from the pressure of the weight. I had officially reached the beached whale stage. Despite how challenging I found a twin pregnancy in the final few weeks, I still miss the magical feeling of my babies kicking and moving inside me. It became increasingly difficult to lift Sophia up onto her changing table and carry her upstairs, so Wes had to take over most of that physical side of parenting. I discovered that wearing a pregnancy belt made a big difference, especially as my bump dropped lower towards the end as the boys moved into the cephalic, or head down, position. One evening when I was about thirty-four weeks pregnant, Wes mused, 'I think it'd be good if they arrived now, because you're really struggling at this point,' but I felt that every single day they spent in the womb would be beneficial to them, as they'd continue to put on more weight, which I thought was a small price to pay for a few weeks of discomfort.

As my due date of 23 November drew near, I began to really look forward to meeting my boys for the first time and holding them. I wondered what they looked like. Would they be completely identical? Perhaps one would have a birthmark or a bit more hair. I was fascinated by my enormous, ever-expanding baby bump and used to lie on the sofa every evening with my hands on my bare bump, just enjoying feeling the boys moving. They were always particularly active when I relaxed. I encouraged Sophia to touch my bump too and explained to her that we would soon be welcoming her two baby brothers into our family. I wondered what she would make of them because she was still a baby herself, and I hoped that she wouldn't be too upset by their arrival. Maybe she'd be fascinated by these two wriggling bundles and they'd play together when the boys were strong enough to sit up by themselves. That would be the perfect ending to our journey, I thought: three happy, healthy children full of energy and fun. I also knew that the minute we laid eyes on them, we'd be completely in love with them, just as we'd been with Sophia.

Everything went smoothly until I went for my routine scan a month before the boys were due to be born and the doctor discovered a degree of placental insufficiency. As he explained, what that meant in my case was that one of the twins might be getting more blood and nutrients than the other. It wasn't alarming at this stage, I was told, as it was still within the normal range, but they'd continue to monitor it. As I was in my final month of pregnancy, I was having weekly scans, and when the next scan indicated normal placental blood flow, I naturally felt huge relief.

On the morning of 17 November, I was due to have a routine scan. I only had six days to go before the birth and I was feeling pretty good. I'd managed to fit in a prenatal workout and the boys were active, wriggling around inside me as much as they could at that stage, so I was happy with their frequency of movement. My hospital bags had been packed for a month and a half and I was feeling well prepared. I drove myself into the city centre for my scan, because Wes wasn't allowed in due to Covid regulations, and settled down on the bed as I usually did. I could sense immediately that something wasn't quite right, as the team conferred, before informing me that the placental resistance they'd spotted a couple of weeks before had returned. Twin two (Oscar) was receiving much higher quantities of blood and nutrients than twin one. Foetal measurements were taken and it appeared that Hugo hadn't grown much in the previous two weeks: while Oscar had gained close to a pound, Hugo had only grown by a couple of ounces. The consultant turned to me and said, 'There's no need to panic because we have it all under control. Their heart rates are normal and there's no sign of distress, but ...' You know when the 'but' comes that it's time to panic. He continued, 'But I want you to go straight home and pack your bags and come in this afternoon. We're going to schedule the delivery for first thing tomorrow morning.' Before I left the hospital, I was given a steroid shot to speed up the boys' lung development, with the second scheduled for later that night.

It was hard to take in. My bags were packed but psychologically I just wasn't prepared. I had been expecting them on Monday 23 November, so it was strange to be told that I'd be having them the very next day. There were only six days in the difference, but at that stage, when you are mentally and physically preparing to have a baby, every day counts. My mind was spinning. All I could think of was that it was Sophia's first birthday that Saturday, 21 November, and I wouldn't be there to celebrate the big day with her. I was so disappointed – she would never turn one again – but felt helpless. The boys needed to be born, and quickly.

Professor Higgins was brilliant at remaining calm and reassuring. 'Just go home and have some lunch. Give Sophia a cuddle and pack your bags and come back in this afternoon.' In a daze, I waddled back to my car, ringing Wes on the way. 'You're never going to believe this, but the boys are coming tomorrow!' He sounded surprised as I quickly explained the situation. Then I left him to absorb the news while I rang my mum, and she was as overwhelmed as I was. But I did what I was told. I went home, threw together a quick bowl of leftovers, went upstairs to pack my last few bits and pieces and then gave Sophia a big hug. I'd prepared two hospital bags, one for myself, with slippers, a dressing-gown, toiletries, an outfit for going home and my hairdryer! Goodness knows how I thought I'd have the time and energy to wash and dry my hair, but I was feeling optimistic. As well as my basics, I'd packed a change or two of pyjamas for each day – ones that buttoned down for breastfeeding, because I planned to do so for at least the first month – as well as fluffy socks and, most importantly, big knickers! Every single one of my friends with children had said to me, 'Whatever you do, don't forget your big Bridget Jones knickers. Buy them in black and make sure they are at least four sizes bigger than your normal size.' I followed their advice. One thoughtful tip that I'd been given, however, was to bring in a nice shower gel for my first shower after the birth to feel that I had a little bit of luxury afterwards. I also packed a silk pillowcase and a silk eye mask to help me sleep. The other bag was for the boys, and I'd been feeling quite pleased with myself that I'd been so well organised with it. I had packed fourteen Ziploc sandwich bags with a little vest, babygro and newborn nappy in each, so that I could just grab one when needed. I also had wipes, soothers, cellular blankets, bibs, muslins, hand sanitiser, nappy bags, nappy cream and various other essentials, but none of the unnecessary extras I'd packed for Sophia. I'd learned that it was best to keep things simple.

Wes and I left at 3.30 that afternoon to drive to the National Maternity Hospital, Holles Street. Thankfully, he was allowed in to help me settle into my room. It was a huge luxury to have a room to myself and I felt very lucky. The team of midwives were so good at helping me to stay calm, checking the babies' heartbeats with a Doppler regularly and keeping my spirits up with a steady supply of tea and encouraging chat. But in spite of their best efforts, it felt surreal to go from anticipating a normal afternoon relaxing at home and playing with Sophia to sitting in a hospital bed, waiting to have a C-section the following day. I looked at my ID wristband and at the two little bands that I'd been given for the boys and thought, *This time tomorrow, I'll be a mum of three.* It was all becoming very real.

Ever since we'd started trying for a family back in 2015, I had been jotting down my favourite baby names and storing them safely in a little notebook. The name Sofia Rose was in there (we later decided to change the spelling), as well as both Hugo and Oscar. Oscar is the name of my mum's maternal grandfather, and we both just really liked the name Hugo. Their middle names are Christopher and Richard, respectively, in homage to their grandfathers. Wes and I had agreed on the names quite early on and love the way they sound together. We didn't tell anyone about our choice, but privately we did call the boys by their names during my pregnancy, which felt like a sweet way to bond with them, especially when I began to feel those exciting first flutters of movement at about eighteen weeks.

I was worried about being away from Sophia for most of the week spent in Holles Street, so I was reassured when Wes rang me on FaceTime that evening so I could say goodnight and blow her a big kiss. Thank goodness for technology. I also had various work commitments to tie up, so I spent an hour emailing and texting, cancelling the last couple of pre-baby appointments with a 'Sorry, but I'm in hospital!' before the midwife came in to say goodnight. 'Try to get some sleep,' she said. 'You've got a big day tomorrow!' Of course, I didn't sleep. When you're heavily pregnant, you have to get up to pee every twenty minutes anyway, but it was also impossible to get comfortable. At home, I had the bed set up with two thick duvets underneath me to ease the pressure on my hips, so I asked for extra pillows and arranged them all around me, with two under my tummy and one under my back, and still I couldn't get to sleep, even with my eye mask. I lay there, thinking about how much my life was going to change in just a few short hours, wondering what it would feel like to hold the boys in my arms for the first time. It was hard to believe that the bump I'd grown so used to over the previous months would soon be two human beings.

My second steroid injection was administered at 2 a.m. and finally, at about 4 a.m., I fell into an uneasy sleep, from which I was awoken by my alarm at 6.30. I knew that I was going to theatre at around 8 a.m., so I had a shower and, because I had time, I decided to put on a bit of make-up to look a little more presentable for meeting my baby boys. A few friends said to me afterwards that they couldn't believe I was wearing make-up in my birth announcement photo, but it was a good distraction. And I needed one because I was already shaking with adrenaline. I really needed Wes's reassurance, but he was driving in from home and had been asked to wait outside until I went into theatre.

Around eight o'clock, there was a light knock on my door and one of the nurses came in saying cheerfully, 'OK, we're going!' The shock of reality set in. This is it, I thought, as we walked slowly towards the lift, this is the moment I've been thinking about for the last eight months and wondering if it would really happen. It had taken a full twenty-eight weeks for me to trust that this pregnancy would last and now, just seven weeks later, I was about to meet my sons for the first time.

'Ready?' the nurse said to me as we moved down the corridor to the operating theatre.

'Ready,' I replied.

I *was* ready, I realised. I had spent the previous half decade of my life trying to have a baby, dealing with the sense of failure, the crushing disappointment that came with every lost pregnancy. Wes and I had had to deal with the fact that our lives might be very different to the ones we had planned: they would involve fun and adventures and hard work, but there would be no children to cuddle and love. Now, in the space of a year, we had found ourselves on a very different path, one that was sometimes scary, worrying and full of

CHAPTER 10

DOUBLE DELIGHT

'd assured the nurse that I was ready, but as soon as I entered the operating theatre, I started to shake uncontrollably. Friends had told me to look out for 'the shakes' but I hadn't expected to feel such a sudden, intense surge of adrenaline. I imagine that when going into labour naturally you have a little more time to process the idea that your baby is going to be born, but with a C-section, it all happens very quickly.

The theatre was bustling with activity as final preparations were made for the surgery. I couldn't speak more highly of the team in Holles Street, led by Professor Higgins. They were kind, reassuring and explained everything clearly to me as it was happening. I was asked to sit on the edge of the operating table while I was given my spinal block. It's similar to an epidural except that it is injected into a slightly different spot in your spine and gives immediate relief, but only lasts for a couple of hours. While we waited for the block to take effect, I made the kind of silly, nervous jokes you make when you are petrified, but everyone worked really hard to make me feel relaxed and comfortable.

With muscles quivering and teeth chattering from the mixture of morphine and adrenaline, I told myself, 'I feel OK, everything will be fine. I feel calm,' but it felt like my whole body was spasming as we waited for the spinal block to work. My legs seemed to turn to jelly, but when they used a cold spray to check if I could feel it, I said, 'Yes, I can,' so they waited a few minutes and tried again. This time, I could feel nothing, and they settled me down for the operation, placing a curtain at chest level. I was trying to focus on taking deep, calming breaths as Wes was brought into the room, beaming. He excitedly squeezed my hand and then he said, 'They've made the first incision!'

'What?' I exclaimed. 'But I didn't feel anything!' I suppose that's the whole point, but I couldn't help thinking that that's why they'd brought Wes in at that very moment – to distract me. Then I felt the tugging sensation, a vigorous pulling and pushing from behind the curtain. As I lay there, I was desperately waiting to hear that first cry because it's seen as a good sign that the lungs are functioning.

The pulling and tugging continued, then Hugo was born first, and as soon as I heard him cry, I started crying. A huge wave of relief and joy surged over me. 'Rosie, he's perfect, he's absolutely perfect,' Wes was saying, tears rolling down his cheeks. As Hugo was the smaller of the twins, I'd been told he might need to go to the neonatal intensive care unit, or NICU. The midwife asked, 'Would you like to hold him first?' Once he had been wiped, weighed and swaddled in a blanket, he was carefully handed to me for some skin-to-skin contact. 'Four pounds seven ounces,' she announced as I looked at his tiny, scrunched-up little face. He was perfect, just as Wes had said. I held him to me, feeling his little heart beating and the warmth of his tiny body, before he was whisked away to the NICU.

Oscar was on the right side of my bump and had been the slightly wilder twin throughout my pregnancy, doing big turns and flips. Now, in the space of time that it took for Hugo to be weighed, Oscar did a back flip in my womb, clearly delighted with all the space to move and stretch now that his brother was gone. The surgeon had to take him out legs first, and as he held him up above the sheet, he did a big wee all over me! That was my introduction to Oscar. He wasn't crying, however, so I panicked for a few seconds before he started to roar. Weighing in at a healthy 5lb 5oz – a good weight for a twin – he was wrapped up in a tiny bundle and handed to me to hold. He was more solid than his brother and a little wriggler, his face scrunching up against the light. He had the tiniest little fingers and toes and little wrinkly knees. To us, he was beautiful.

The whole operation was over surprisingly quickly. Apart from the shakes and meeting my two gorgeous baby boys for the first time, one of my lasting memories of the C-section was the feeling of being empty and my organs settling back into their original position. They'd been so squashed during my pregnancy that it felt lovely to have some room again. I was stitched up, wheeled into the recovery room and handed a glass of water, which felt unbelievably good to drink. A little while later, back in my room, I was given manna from heaven in the form of tea and toast. There's truly nothing like it. White toast with one of those little pots of raspberry jam – what could be nicer? I was ravenous, having fasted from nine o'clock the previous evening, so it was absolutely delicious.

Oscar was whisked away to the NICU soon after Hugo, as he was struggling to breathe properly. His breathing problems were due to amniotic fluid on his lungs, so they put him on a machine called CPAP. This means continuous positive airway pressure and allows the patient to breathe better. In fact, it has been used for Covid patients and it's also used to treat sleep apnoea. I squeezed Wes's hand really tightly and asked the midwife how serious it was, but she reassured me that Oscar would be fine with a little bit of help from the experienced team in the neonatal department.

I vaguely recall lying in the recovery room, excitedly texting family and friends with the good news that the twins had been safely born, and thinking that I felt pretty good. I'd had very little time to tell anyone that I was going into hospital, so it felt wonderful to tell everyone our big news.

Looking back, though, I can see that I was far from normal. I was coming down from painkillers and morphine, not to mention the spinal block, and in a matter of minutes, I'd become a mum to twins. I felt as if I was drunk or something!

I spent about an hour in recovery being monitored, and my wound was checked again before I was wheeled back to my hospital room and transferred into bed. It felt a little bit disconcerting, however, to be without the babies beside me in their little cots. I'd imagined them side by side, as they had been in my womb, and now I felt as if I'd barely met them before they'd been whisked away. It seemed surreal, as if I hadn't really given birth to them. But a couple of hours later, one of the midwives came in and asked Wes and me if we'd like to go down to the NICU and see the twins.

I was gently helped into a wheelchair and Wes wheeled me down to the unit to meet our boys. I peered in at them in their incubators and it came as a shock to see just how tiny they were. Sophia had been born full term, and even though she'd only been 6lb 8oz, which I'd consider small, she'd looked like a giant compared to them. They looked so fragile, with their little stick legs and tiny feet and hands, I could hardly believe it. *Oh my goodness*, I thought, as I looked at each twin, *did this person just come from me?* It felt strange to think that these human beings had been growing inside me for most of the year, and that I was meeting them properly for the first time. I was lucky to be able to cuddle Hugo, because Oscar was still on the CPAP machine, lying on his little tummy, and we have a lovely photo of him between his proud mum and dad. I'm smiling with joy in the picture, but I do look as overwhelmed and exhausted as I felt, while Wes sports a huge, happy grin. Our family was complete.

By 4 p.m., Wes had to go home to Sophia and I was wheeled back into my room. It felt very strange to be there by myself. The cots had been removed and their hospital bag remained unopened on the floor. I couldn't help but wonder if the past twenty-four hours had actually happened. After a bite to eat, I slipped on my eye mask, propped myself sideways on the pillows to find a comfortable position without disturbing my incision site, and managed to nod off. It felt so different to that first night with Sophia, where I'd lain awake until the early hours, watching her little chest rise and fall with every breath. Even though the circumstances of the twins' birth were very different, I felt more relaxed knowing that at least I had an idea of what life with a small baby would entail. Now, all I had to do was to work out what life with two small babies and a toddler would be like ...

I was woken some hours later by a light tap on my arm. I lifted my eye mask to see one of the midwives on duty smiling down at me. 'I brought you a cup of tea, and I need you to produce some colostrum for the boys,' she said gently. Colostrum is what is produced before breast milk; it's incredibly rich, full of antibodies and offers immune support, so it would be a huge benefit to the boys. The only problem was, I didn't know how to produce it. 'I'm sorry,' I said, 'I've never expressed by hand or even breastfed before.' She helped and showed me how to express the colostrum into a syringe and, once again, I was amazed by what my own body is capable of. I never imagined that I'd be able to grow and feed my own babies. The midwife removed the catheter from my bladder and suggested I take a shower. Those of you who have had a C-section will know that standing up for the first time afterwards is a pretty bizarre feeling. I felt woozy and lightheaded as I half-stumbled towards the bathroom. I was so sweaty and sticky that it was a relief to have a long, hot shower.

The first glimpse of my post-partum body came as a shock. Mum had warned me in advance. 'You're not going to like your tummy straight after birth. Take it from me, it'll look like jelly.' To me, it looked like a golf ball in a sock! I stood in amazement looking at myself in the mirror, so swollen from fluid retention, with my soft, sagging tummy, but I wasn't disgusted by any means. I was incredibly proud of what remained of my enormous baby bump and all that my body had managed to achieve over the past eight months. I knew that my little pot belly wouldn't last forever but, for now, it was a reminder of what I'd been through and wanted for so long. I cautiously inspected my incision site, which was much smaller and neater than I'd anticipated. It was hard to believe that two little humans had emerged through it earlier that day.

I pulled on a clean pair of pyjamas after my shower, settled into bed and went back to sleep, ready to be woken in another three hours to express more colostrum. I was told that by the third day my milk would come in and then I'd be able to express, or even breastfeed if the babies were able to latch on. I didn't realise that this would be the toughest part of my stay in hospital. Friends of mine who've had babies say that it takes time for breastfeeding to become established, and I found it very hard because I didn't have the boys with me in the room. I also missed Sophia terribly, and even though Wes rang me every night so that I could say goodnight to her on FaceTime, I wasn't at home being her mum – or caring for the boys, because they were downstairs being looked after 24/7 by the incredible team in the NICU. I was all alone in my little nest, without my chicks.

Thankfully, the hospital has lactation consultants on hand to give advice and support on breastfeeding and mine suggested looking at the boys' clothes or thinking about them, but I found it all incredibly stressful. I set my alarm for every three hours, and during the daytime, I'd go downstairs to feed the boys myself. I was thrilled when Hugo, the smaller twin, managed to latch on, but because he was tiny, he found it too difficult in the end, so the team advised me to try expressing milk to feed to them in a small bottle. A hospital-grade breast pump was wheeled into my room and I'd spend about ten minutes at a time double expressing, feeling like a cow in the milking shed. I was quite successful at it, which made me feel a bit better. I was also reassured that I'd be able to keep an eye on the volume that the boys were getting from the bottle, so I'd know that they were feeding well and getting the nutrition they needed. I stopped feeling guilty about it then because I thought that the most important thing was that they get my breast milk, in whatever form it came, for as long as I could manage, even if it was only a few weeks.

The next few days in hospital passed in a blur of expressing and feeding, eating and sleeping when I possibly could, but there was no sense of routine or rhythm and I began to feel that familiar tightness at the base of my skull that told me I was getting a stress headache. At first, I thought it was due to the anaesthetic and I texted Professor Higgins to ask, 'I'm getting these awful headaches – could they be connected in any way to the spinal block?' He did a neurological exam on me to ensure that there was no connection between the spinal block and my headaches and concluded that there wasn't. They were simply down to lack of sleep and stress, despite how kind and supportive the midwives looking after me were. But I put a huge amount of pressure on myself and I'm conscious as I write this that it may sound as if I'm complaining, but I'm really not. I was over the moon to be a mum of three after all that we'd been through. I knew that this unsettled period would soon end, and I couldn't wait to take the boys home to Sophia so that we could begin life as a family of five.

One feeling that took me by surprise was guilt. As Sophia's birthday passed, on the Saturday of my week in hospital, I felt a deep sense of sadness that I hadn't been able to give birth to my beautiful baby girl. I kept trying to rationalise it and reason with myself that we went through so much to have her and that we were incredibly lucky that our surrogacy journey had been such a success, but I couldn't help feeling intense guilt that I was able to give birth to the boys but wasn't able to give birth to her. I was also heartbroken that I was in hospital and couldn't be home for her birthday. I knew that she was too young to understand the difference, but it mattered to me.

Later that afternoon, Mum rang me as she did every day during my hospital stay because she wasn't allowed to visit me due to Covid restrictions. 'Do you feel tearful at all?' she asked carefully. I did because of Sophia's birthday, not for the reasons she'd expected – the low mood that some women experience around day three after giving birth when there's a shift in hormone levels. 'I'm actually in pretty good spirits,' I said gratefully. The only real experience I had of a hormone shift was a bout of night sweats on that third night after the birth, but otherwise I managed to avoid the baby blues. A shower and a change of pyjamas sorted the night sweats out, and once I had worked through my guilty feelings about missing Sophia's birthday, I felt very upbeat and positive for the rest of the week. The boys were doing well and improving every day, which made me feel much more confident and relaxed. They did have to have photo-therapy for jaundice, just as Sophia had done, but apart from that, they were feeding well and growing increasingly alert considering their gestational age. Both continued to drink my expressed breast milk, in addition to being fed via an IV drip, and I had grown accustomed to expressing every three hours. Before being cleared to leave hospital, they were given a range of routine tests for eyesight, hearing and signs of hip dysplasia and blood tests to show that their jaundice had resolved. All were clear. Soon, they'd be ready to go home.

I was discharged from hospital on Monday 23 November, two days before the boys. It was actually my original due date, but it felt as if a lifetime had passed. Packing up my bags, I felt such a wave of relief that I had given birth a few days earlier than planned and the twins had arrived into the world safely.

I was a little emotional saying goodbye to the wonderful team of midwives, as I'd grown so fond of them all and was grateful for the support and advice they'd given me, particularly when I was struggling in the first few days. Wes collected me from hospital, and as we travelled home through the sunny Dublin streets, I tried to imagine how our lives would be as parents of three. My mum was playing with Sophia in the garden when we arrived back at the house, and I was so excited to finally cuddle my little girl. I couldn't believe how much she'd changed in the short time that I'd been away. When I'd left for hospital, she was a baby, and when I came home, she was a toddler. I'm used to spending all day with my children, so I don't necessarily notice them growing, but after just a week, she really felt different. I could see that her little teeth had grown and I spotted the first signs of her toddler tantrums! I hadn't anticipated that she'd develop so much in that short space of time, and I was surprised that she seemed a little bit strange with me, not as affectionate as before or interested in being around me. Puzzled, I asked Wes, 'Am I imagining it or is Sophia being weird with me?'

'I haven't noticed,' he said. 'She seems fine.' It was only later that he admitted that, yes, she had been a bit disinterested. She had grown used to her dad and my mum looking after her, changing her and feeding her, and now I had returned, expecting everything to be normal. It was hard to accept that she was so annoyed with me for leaving her, but at the same time, I found it amazing that she was now becoming her own little person. I had found it upsetting towards the end of my pregnancy that I simply couldn't carry Sophia around any more, take her for walks, give her baths or carry her upstairs to bed, and after my C-section I had to be extremely careful to avoid lifting. So, while I still couldn't fully care for Sophia, I made it up to her at mealtimes and with plenty of cuddles and fun.

The next two days disappeared in a blur of activity as we prepared our house for the boys' homecoming. We set up a pair of cots downstairs and upstairs for day- and night-time, although the twins were small enough to safely share a cot downstairs for the first few weeks. Wes finished putting them together, watched inquisitively by Sophia, while I carefully sterilised bottles and teats, arranged their size zero nappies on the changing table beside packets of wipes and cotton wool and folded their tiny newborn vests into drawers. We also visited the boys in hospital and I brought in bottles of my freshly expressed breast milk, carefully packed into an insulated cool-bag. Before we brought them home, the wonderful team in the NICU at Holles Street gave us a detailed briefing on caring for premature babies, including safety and hygiene advice, sleeping arrangements, milk volumes to aim for at each feed and recommendations for reducing risks associated with cot death, or SIDS. We were given a prescription for an infant iron supplement, vitamin D drops and a post-discharge premature infant formula. Later on, we also needed medication for reflux.

Then it was time to make one final drive to the hospital to pick them up. I was feeling very emotional that day as we said goodbye to the team, who'd looked after them so well, and tucked the boys into their car seats. They looked so tiny, snuggled up fast asleep under cosy blankets, ready to travel home to meet their big sister and begin their lives with us as a family of five.

Walking into our house with the twins for the first time was a special, unforgettable moment. Mum and Dad were there with Sophia, who stared wide-eyed in surprise at these two sleepy little figures lying side by side in the cot in our kitchen. Wes's parents joined us, and as we introduced them to their new grandchildren, there were a few tears of joy and relief that they were home safely. Everyone was amazed at how small they were, as the photos I had sent from hospital didn't fully show their tiny stick legs and delicate features. They could hardly believe that, despite being born at just thirty-six weeks, they were perfectly able to feed and breathe. They were surprisingly alert, waking up to take in their new surroundings. It's amazing how tough little babies can be. Sophia was fascinated by her twin brothers. She reached out to touch their hands and smiled down at them while we explained that they were the very same two people who had been inside Mummy's tummy for the previous few months. But the novelty quickly wore off as a nearby toy seemed more appealing. Later that day, I noticed that she wasn't looking quite as pleased with them. I could almost see her thoughts: *I can't play with them, I can't eat them – what's their purpose? They're taking all of Mum and Dad's atten-tion and all they do is cry.*

Bringing the boys home was a poignant moment because it felt like the closure of a difficult chapter in our lives and the opening of another. We'd gone from a couple struggling to have a baby to a family of five in the space of a couple of years. There was such a satisfying feeling of completion to it, with our three healthy children. I felt a wave of relief to be free from the worries and stresses that come with fertility issues: the uncertainty and frustration of infertility and the heartbreak of miscarriages. It felt liberating to be able to move forward with our lives and look forward to watching our children grow up together.

CHAPTER 11

WORKING MUM

I t's difficult to describe how chaotic and intense life can be with three babies who are close in age. Partly, this was because Wes and I had decided that we'd try to do everything ourselves, with a little help from our mums. I don't know what we were thinking! Sophia was still waking during the night and the boys needed to be fed every three hours, so on our first night home we got twenty minutes' sleep. The second night, we managed a blissful half an hour, and by the third, we looked at each other and said, 'We can't do this!' We were grey with exhaustion and I was trying to cope with recovering from my C-section, a serious operation. Both boys had developed symptoms of reflux and colic within the first week of arriving home, so feeding them became a lengthy process of winding them thoroughly and keeping them upright for as long as possible before putting them down to sleep. My consultant had written me a prescription for Losec, a type of proton-pump inhibitor to help reduce the amount of acid produced in the stomach. We also used infant microbiotics, lactose drops and simethicone. We couldn't take turns with the feeding while the other had a sleep because we had a baby each. Mum was a brilliant support, coming over to our house every afternoon and urging us to go upstairs for a nap, but half an hour just wasn't enough to refresh us. The exhaustion was relentless.

Some of you might well say, 'What did you expect?' but I don't think anything quite prepares you for life with three babies of one and under, all of whom have the same needs at more or less the same time. I was trying not to complain about something that we'd wanted for so long. I felt that I wasn't in a position to give out about anything when there were so many people out there desperate to have a baby. But while Wes and I put on a smile, drank a lot of coffee and joked about feeling constantly 'stunned', the exhaustion was wearing us down. The advice is always 'sleep when the baby sleeps', but when do you get the laundry done, prepare the dinner and look after an energetic toddler? I still needed to give Sophia three nourishing meals a day, plus plenty of snacks to keep her energy levels up. We were officially outnumbered. This was November/December 2020 during the Covid-19 pandemic, and the resulting lockdowns and restrictions on visitors to homes meant that we couldn't have extra people in the house.

Our recent experience with Sophia as a newborn had helped us to feel a lot more confident with feeding, changing and interpreting cries, and our house was very much set up for babies, with four changing tables dotted around between upstairs and downstairs. I found it easier to express breast milk when I was home taking care of the boys, but it soon became clear that I wasn't eating enough or getting enough rest to be able to produce milk in the quantities they increasingly required. Friends have told me that breastfeeding just one baby is incredibly time-consuming, and I discovered that expressing the milk and feeding them every three hours had to be carefully planned out. Wes and I used to sit on the sofa with a baby each and laugh at ourselves – I think we were hysterical from sleep deprivation. When you have a baby, there are also so many emotions to reconcile and understand as a parent: happiness and gratitude, of course, but also feeling down sometimes due to lack of sleep and dealing with guilt. I wanted to be there for everyone: to play with Sophia, bathe her and feed her, to be there for the boys who needed me so much and to also be emotionally available to support Wes. I was putting a lot of pressure on myself to look after everyone, and that was even more exhausting.

In hindsight, Christmas was quite funny. For a start, most of it is a blur. We decided to have my parents and brother and sister-in-law to our house, because it would mean that we wouldn't have to pack three babies, two dogs and everything they needed into the car and drive to Wicklow. Dad had come up with the bright idea of having dinner catered and had organised the food weeks in advance. We dragged ourselves up on Christmas Day after two hours of sleep. I changed and dressed Sophia, brought her downstairs to make her breakfast and somehow managed to put on a smart dress, having washed and dried my hair the night before. Mum had brought everything to set the Christmas table and arranged it the previous day, adding candles and a festive centrepiece. We fed the boys just before the food was ready and, by some miracle, they slept soundly while we ate Christmas dinner with Sophia beside us in her high chair. But by five o'clock, Wes and I felt delirious with tiredness and I began to giggle hysterically at everything, so we were sent off like small children to have a nap.

Dad had urged me to consider getting a night nurse but I was reluctant, feeling that if I wanted to be a mum to them, that meant doing it all. Why do we mothers do this to ourselves? The reality quickly dawned on me that I'd have to put guilt aside and accept help before Wes and I lost our minds due to sleep deprivation. Thankfully, a friend of mine recommended a night nurse, who was available to come in every second night, so we could look forward to having more sleep. We stopped trying to do it all ourselves, and having the support made a huge difference to our mental, emotional and physical health. The nurse also planned to sleep train the twins, so that eventually they'd sleep through the night for us.

What might seem like a luxury to some was a necessity to us, but it's not cheap and we needed to have a plan to pay for her help. Wes's business had been closed for most of the previous year so we decided that I'd go back to work, after taking just a few weeks off for maternity leave, and accept the various work offers and opportunities that presented themselves. It was really tough, but being self-employed, maternity leave is an ideal rather than a reality. I'm fortunate to be able to monetise my online platform, which allows me to work from home, therefore it made sense to swap roles. Wes is a brilliant dad and more than happy to do his share of nappy changing and feeding and, although he misses running the business, it worked well for both of us. I'd say that this was a common scenario for couples during the pandemic. It wasn't necessarily what I wanted, but gradually I grew accustomed to it and even enjoyed my little virtual outings to the adult world.

In order to be work ready, I was keen to build my strength and fitness again. Recovery after a C-section is gradual, so I couldn't rush it, and I was quite proud of my postpartum bump anyway. It showed that I'd just given birth to two babies, which for me was a huge achievement. One night just a few days after we brought the boys home from hospital, I remember twisting awkwardly in bed to pick up Hugo out

I've always been focused on my fitness and have found it to be essential for stress relief. Time spent in the gym, out for a run or at a Pilates class is important for releasing endorphins, clearing your head and boosting mental clarity, and I was keen to return to my training regime as soon as I was allowed to. I knew that I needed to relax for the first few weeks and allow my body to heal, but at my six-week check-up my GP advised that I could return to light exercise, such as walking locally in the park with the pushchair and gentle mat Pilates exercises. After my twelve-week check-up with Professor Higgins, I was allowed to go back to weight training. I started with light weights, building from there, and my strength gradually returned. Most days, I managed to squeeze in a 30–45 minute workout and I followed a programme designed by my personal trainer based on two upper-body and two lower-body resistance-training days a week, plus regular cardio and core exercises. You really can't rush postpartum exercise for your abs, though, and I focused on building them up slowly and safely, concentrating on engaging my deep core muscles. It was a really enjoyable process, because I love feeling strong and fit, and my home workouts have probably helped to keep me relatively sane.

Indeed, health, fitness and nutrition have always been a passion and an important part of my life, going right back to primary school where my interest in athletics, hockey and tennis began. My favourite subject in school was biology, especially human physiology. I used to represent Leinster in

100m hurdles and high jump competitions and trained with an athletics club, so I made sure to eat a diet that properly supported my fitness and activity levels. My mum grows her own fresh organic produce, so I was brought up to appreciate the many benefits of homegrown, seasonal food.

I've always found that one of the most effective ways to keep fit and stay consistently active is to make exercise a normal part of my lifestyle. It's as much a part of my daily routine now as having a shower or brushing my teeth. This way, I view it as a lifestyle and time out to destress rather than a punishment. A combination of resistance training with weights, Pilates and cardiovascular exercise suits me best and I used to love running but now prefer exercise that is gentler on joints. But no matter how disciplined and determined you may be, it's very difficult to motivate yourself to get active when it's something you don't enjoy, and in my experience, exercise should be fun, challenging and changed up regularly to make sure it never gets boring. Discover which activity works best for you and always pay attention to your body's sometimes subtle signals. Make sure you get sufficient downtime, and if you're feeling tired or sore, prioritise rest and relaxation to avoid a potential injury. Jogging, gardening, cycling, dancing, yoga, sea swimming and power walking with a pushchair are great examples of fun and free activities. Indeed, I started with short gentle walks pushing the double pram with Hugo and Oscar once I was given the go-ahead to build up my fitness again. To benefit the most from it, aim to get your heart rate up during exercise, challenge your body and get a little out of breath.

There have been plenty of days since Sophia and the twins were born when a home workout is the last thing I want to do, and lying on the sofa with a cup of tea during their nap time is far more appealing than lifting weights or sweating on a cardio machine. But as most of us know, the benefits of an active lifestyle go far beyond aesthetics. I love the physical strength, good mood, boosted energy levels, focus on healthy eating, improved sleep and stronger immune system that regular exercise gives me. Furthermore, I've always found weight training to be most effective for sculpting your body, improving the muscle to fat ratio, and it's particularly important for supporting bone health in women. I aim to incorporate resistance training into my workouts two to four times a week, depending on my energy levels, and I adapt my sessions to how I'm feeling, always listening to my body.

For the majority of people, the most intimidating aspect of embarking on a new fitness regime is simply where to begin. It can sometimes feel like the media is constantly bombarding us with conflicting information and the latest findings about nutrition, fat loss and fitness, making it extremely challenging for a novice to know where to start and how to design meals and supplements to support their fitness goals. If your aim is to build muscle or lose body fat, then your approach to nutrition must reflect that, otherwise your exercise efforts may be wasted. However, I'm a big believer in keeping your fitness and eating plans as simple and achievable as possible. Life can be complicated enough without adding further unnecessary stresses! It's important to focus on making small changes that will fit in with your lifestyle and be sustainable. A complete lifestyle overhaul isn't practical for everyone, and life inevitably gets in the way, so taking it in baby steps and always moving in the right direction is the best way to make sustainable healthy changes. Most importantly, do what works for you. If you're a member of a gym or other sports club, don't be afraid to ask fitness experts as many questions as you need to because that's what they're there for.

If you're struggling to find the motivation to exercise regularly, I've discovered that having colourful, functional and fun workout clothes to wear can help to give me the boost I need on low-energy days, and a decent pair of runners will make all the difference to your training experience and may even help to prevent an injury.

Building awareness around food and fitness and practising mindful eating are key to avoiding overindulging, although it tends to be individual to all of us. For example, I aim to eat until I'm three-quarters full, and I focus on filling up with salad or vegetables first. For others, it could be swapping bread for a wrap, sweetened cereal for porridge, avoiding alcohol on weekdays, drinking water instead of a soft drink, going to the gym or a fitness class two or three times a week, taking less sugar in your tea or coffee or enjoying a piece of fresh fruit instead of a chocolate bar. I know that lots of us are driven by an upcoming holiday, wedding, significant birthday or event and hope to feel confident in a special outfit, so having a fitness, health or weight goal in mind is often the best motivation. Visualise how you want to look and feel and aim for your lifestyle and every health-related decision you make to support your vision. Another powerful motivator is accountability. Consider asking a friend with similar goals to be a fitness buddy to go for brisk walks or to gym classes with you. You're more likely to stick to a fitness plan if you're helping to support each other, and plenty of gyms, sports clubs and trainers offer classes specifically for mums and babies, tailored to support the important post-partum stage.

As a mother, following a healthy lifestyle has played just as important a role in my everyday routine as it always did because it has been my experience that taking the time during a busy day with children to get some exercise and make positive choices around food, stress management and snacking can have a big impact on the kind of parent you are. I have discovered that I'm more energetic, fun and patient as a mum when I've had the chance to go out for a walk with the pushchair or train in our small home gym, even for just thirty minutes a day. It's the only time out of twenty-four hours that I'm not on call, that I can switch off and enjoy silence or listen to a podcast. Wes and I take it in turns to mind the babies while the other works out, although we do

I'm very much aware that not everybody is as fortunate as we have been, and many couples are forced to abandon their family dreams for financial reasons or because they've run out of options and don't have the mental or emotional energy to continue fighting. I completely understand that and I've been close to that point. But if you do have a successful conclusion to your journey and your much-longed-for baby arrives safely into your arms, then you may feel, as I did at the start, that you must dedicate your entire existence to this tiny human and allow your own needs to fade into the background. When the twins were born, I knew more about what to anticipate with newborn life and how to be a present, contented parent. Despite how incredibly busy those early days with the boys were, when they fed every three hours and struggled with colic and reflux, I found that I still remained mindful about my own health and self-care needs. To me, they were simply a job requirement and non-negotiable. No matter how exhausted I felt, I made sure to shower and get dressed each day and make healthy food choices – most of the time. I enjoyed indulging in veggie pizzas and sausages late at night when we didn't have the energy to throw together even a basic meal, but generally I ate nutritious food and plenty of quick, easy smoothies with big handfuls of dark leafy greens to help support my energy levels postpartum. Mum was amazing too, bringing over huge pots of soup, vegetable stews and quinoa dishes to keep us well fed. Once my doctor gave me permission, I without realising it and eventually had to wean myself off, so I would love to advise my teenage self to eat a sensible, balanced diet with regular meals and snacks to avoid binge-ing. These days, I mostly avoid refined sugar completely, as it really doesn't agree with me and makes me feel very jittery. As a new parent, the quick energy rush that refined sugar can give you is extremely tempting, and it can be very difficult to focus on your health when there are so many new and unprecedented demands being made on your energy and time. Babies are, by their very nature, highly unpredicta-ble and – as many of us are aware! – their sleep patterns are too. Yet small changes can make a big difference to new parents trying to navigate life with a newborn and, as I discovered, can support your patience and understand-ing in more testing moments. I would encourage people to start off by making small changes, such as swapping their chocolate bar or packet of crisps for a piece of whole fruit. Buying whole, fresh and unprocessed foods is important too, as it helps to wean you off the taste of sugar and salt-rich processed ingredients. Staying active and drinking plenty of water all make a big difference. Education is key too, and it helps people to avoid being convinced by clever market-ing to buy health products lacking convincing research to support their efficacy. I'm a big advocate of intuitive eating and mindful eating because listening to your body's hunger signals is such an important aspect of healthy living. We're all biochemically, genetically and metabolically individual, overall mood and motivation. I overhauled my diet about ten years ago by mostly eliminating processed foods and refined sugar and really increasing my consumption of plant-based whole foods. I couldn't believe the difference in how I felt in just a few short weeks. My sleep and recovery from workouts improved, my energy levels soared and my skin looked better too. It's important to make positive health and lifestyle choices if you want to look and feel your best. Yet many people are reluctant to make the necessary changes for a healthier lifestyle, and it can become even more difficult when you have children. Lack of knowledge on how to make positive dietary choices is certainly one of the reasons, but food is also very personal and influenced by emotions, cultural preferences, family traditions, taste preferences, nostalgia. Significantly changing your diet and approach to eating can be a huge challenge for multiple reasons, but making small changes can make a big difference – especially swapping processed food for real food and sugar-laden juice or fizzy drinks for cold-pressed vegetable juice, simple water or caffeine-free herbal teas. Furthermore, I believe that optimising digestive well-being can benefit skin, hair and immune system health. We're not what we eat, we're what we absorb! Working to support digestive health encourages optimal absorption of the key nutrients needed for every metabolic function, and a diet rich in a wide variety of plant fibres, plus regular consumption of probiotic and prebiotic foods, can really benefit digestive health. I've been taking probiotics for the past six or seven years to support normal digestive health and optimise nutrient absorption, which I find also benefits my energy levels, skin, digestion and immune system health. Part of my MSc dissertation focused on the benefits of EPA and DHA essential fatty acids, and in addition to iron and folic acid, I was careful to include it as a supplement throughout my pregnancy. If you're vegan or don't like the taste of fish, an algae-based omega-3 may be important for ensuring you get sufficient levels of long-chain poly-unsaturated fatty acids EPA and DHA to support normal cell membrane function and structure and cardiovascular, brain and joint health. I also strongly recommend that vegans take a daily B12 supplement to prevent a deficiency, as it's one of the only nutrients that's difficult to obtain from plant-based foods.

From speaking to hundreds of people about healthier living over the past few years, when I ran a number of health and fitness workshops across Ireland to tie in with the release of my cookbooks, one theme has consistently cropped up when they talk about trying to make more positive food choices: how little time they have to actually shop for and prepare food – particularly if you're a working parent, as I've discovered. I've always enjoyed cooking, baking and making favourite meals and snacks at home, but during the latter part of my pregnancy I found it difficult to stand up for more than ten or fifteen minutes before I began to feel tired and sore. Since the twins have arrived, I've struggled to find the time to cook beyond what I make for Sophia, and I often find myself batch cooking and freezing meals or relying on foods that are quick, easy and nourishing. Many of us lead busy, demanding lives and need simple, nutritious meal and snack ideas with ingredients that don't cost huge amounts and can be easily sourced in most shops and supermarkets.

Throughout the pandemic lockdowns of 2020 and 2021, Wes and I relied on home-delivery shopping services for much of our food and household essentials. Not only are they really convenient when you have a busy home to run and very limited time between various baby feeds to go any-where, I also find that I make fewer impulse buys and spend less money than when I go to a supermarket. Aside from fresh produce, I stocked up on beans, pulses, dried grains, herbs, spices, sauces, nuts, seeds and nut butters for quick, healthy meals and snacks. I love oatcakes with almond butter or hummus for a simple, satisfying snack and Sophia has recently been enjoying them spread with organic peanut butter. I've discovered over the past year and a half that the trick to ensuring she sleeps through the night is to encour-age her to eat filling and nourishing meals and snacks. So I find foods like avocado, nut butter, cheese and porridge really beneficial for her. Of course, she loves baby biscuits and tasty treats too, but she knows that she can only enjoy them after she's eaten her meal.

For quick smoothies to make in the morning and bring out with you, a favourite tip of mine is to divide fruit and veg ingredients into freezer bags in advance to freeze and have on hand. Then simply add your liquid base and any other fillers you like, such as nuts, seeds, nut butters, protein powders or oats to whizz up a more satisfying smoothie. Indeed, frozen fruit and vegetables are a useful option when under time pressure. I often use frozen berries, bananas, pineapple, kale and spinach for smoothies and peas, sweetcorn, carrot and green beans to add to stews, soups and vegetable curries. Easy, nutritious food doesn't take hours to prepare, especially when you aim to keep some fresh vegetables and sources of protein in the fridge and non-perishable items in your cupboards, including foods like quinoa, rice, pasta and canned beans.

Indeed, I've discovered that my time-management skills in both family food prep and my professional life have improved a lot now that I'm a mum of three. Once we decided that I'd go back to work, I quickly had to get used to finding windows of opportunity to take a picture or an interview for a brand ambassador partnership, carving out time between naps and feeding or when Mum came over to take the boys or Sophia out for a walk in their pushchairs. I've worked for myself since I was nineteen so I'm sort of conditioned not to turn down jobs or work opportunities – it seems to be part of the deal when you're a freelancer, even though Wes and my parents often tell me to just relax and not to work every spare moment I have. But somehow I find a way to fit it in, and I prefer to be kept busy. It does suit me to multitask, to take on different projects and have different elements to my life – it keeps my easily bored mind occupied.

Despite the many challenges of juggling family life with three very young children and going back to work so soon after giving birth, I feel incredibly grateful that we've managed to establish a routine and sense of balance, with plenty of help and support from our respective families. I was lucky to have been in a position to return to working from home in the midst of a global pandemic and it's taught me a lot about how to best manage my time and energy levels. And parenting feels more natural and less overwhelming than when Sophia was a newborn. With each new developmental phase that Sophia, Hugo and Oscar move into and as their ability to communicate their needs improves too, we feel increasingly confident and reassured that we can cope with everything.

CHAPTER 12

WES AND ME PLUS THREE

Since having children, a lot of people have said to me, 'Enjoy the baby phase. It flies by so quickly.' By seven o'clock in the evening, after a long day of feeding, soothing and changing nappy explosions, when the boys are both roaring with teething pain and Sophia is grizzling with tiredness, I have to admit that I sometimes think it's going on for far too long. Occasionally, in the sheer chaos of life with three babies, I have to remind myself that this is what I've always wanted.

Having twins has been challenging, rewarding and seriously intense! We thought we had plenty of experience with babies after having Sophia, but there has already been so much to learn about the boys and all of their little idiosyncrasies. It amazes me that, with the same genetic material, the boys have different personalities, likes and dislikes. We fondly call Hugo 'Party Boy H' because he's always the last one to settle down to bed and loves to be part of the action, watching his sister run around the kitchen. He has a charming smile, a cheeky giggle and a glint in his eye. I joke that he wants to sneak out to Coppers nightclub when we're all asleep. Oscar is more laid-back and loves his grub but also enjoys watching the hubbub of activity at home. He has a big, beautiful smile that will undoubtedly break a few hearts in the future. Both boys are already great fun, always smiling big gurgly grins and trying desperately to sit up by themselves. They love music and being sung to – you wouldn't believe the tuneless singing that goes on in the house. 'How Much is That Doggy in the Window?' is a catchy number, and 'Incy Wincy Spider', 'The Teddy Bears' Picnic' and 'The Bear Went Over the Mountain' are all classics that they adore. I can already tell we are going to have such fun with them and can imagine all the mischief they'll get up to with their big sister leading the way.

Wes and I are also fascinated by how they connect. We have a twin feeding chair in the kitchen, and we'll sit them up beside each other in that and facing each other in their baby play gym. They'll smile and chat together, little coos and babbles and giggles. We joke that they have their own secret language and they seem so in sync. If one cries, the

We're also having great fun watching Sophia grow into her role as a big sister to the boys. We enjoyed our time with her so much as a family of three during the lockdowns of 2020, and part of me does miss that, but we're proud parents watching her change and grow from baby to child, learning to walk and saying new words. She points at the sky and says 'birr' for birds, while dogs are 'wawa' and she says 'numnum' when she's hungry or asking for a snack. She says 'hiya' to everyone and my dad gets a special 'hi grandpa' greeting from her. Often we hear her repeat words or phrases she's heard earlier that day or week, and it amazes me how much she listens to us. She's getting much more confident about communicating with us, although I suspect she understand far more than we even realise. For the first couple of months, Sophia was unsure about the twins, even a little jealous when she saw us feeding them, but now she's become much more accepting of them. She sees them as interesting little people because they're much more communicative. She'll run over to them in their twin chair to chat to them, give them a little cuddle and try to share her snacks. I've found her offering Oscar some of her crunchy biscuits, with a cheeky grin. His eyes were wide with temptation, but we're only beginning to offer them solids like baby rice and purees. It's wonderful to see her really interacting with them now. Having the twins has changed the household dynamic in such an enjoyable way and I'm so pleased that Sophia has the boys' company. I found it sad that living through the pandemic meant Sophia couldn't play with other babies and toddlers. I know she's still only little, but that interaction is so important, I think. I have lots of friends with babies of her age, but we haven't been able to get together and really enjoy those outings to the park. Mum reassures me that, because she's still so young, she'll be able to catch up, but I often think about how the pandemic has affected our children. We've had our precious family time, but they are really losing out in many respects. Thankfully, we are lucky enough to have a nice garden for Sophia to explore every day, with the boys in their double pushchair, and we bring her out for walks most days, so she gets a lot of outdoor time, just like I did when I was growing up. We're lucky enough to have a lovely local park with a big playground and we enjoy bringing the children there when the weather is fine. Sophia loves going down the slide, with the twins watching from their pushchair.

I'm also becoming more confident in my life as a working mum and have become an excellent scheduler. A friend will see a post of mine on social media or note my involvement in a campaign and say, 'How did you find time to do that?' It's literally because I have built everything I have to do work-wise into the golden hour in the early afternoon when they are all napping and any other little pockets of time that I find. I've become very resourceful and don't waste a minute of the day. If I have to take a photo for a work commitment, I'll wash my hair the night before and during a ten-minute window, just after I've given Sophia her bowl of porridge for breakfast, I'll do my make-up while she munches on a piece of toast or a few slices of peeled apple. It's amazing what you can squeeze into a few minutes, I find. I'll bet most parents feel the same. They use the word 'juggling' for a reason!

If I don't have any work commitments or Zoom meetings, I'm very casually dressed at home with the kids, in a pair of leggings and oversize hoodie, because there's no time to put on anything else. Although the boys have started weaning, they still have five bottle feeds in twenty-four hours, so life is a constant blur of feeding times, nappy changes, playtime, laundry – so much laundry! – and keeping the house relatively clean. Standards have definitely fallen when it comes to domestic tasks like cooking meals for me and Wes, but I'm very conscious of keeping the floor clean because Sophia, being a typical toddler, will drop food on it and pick it up again to eat. In fact, her favourite game is to 'feed' our two little Pomeranians, dropping food down to them and watching them gobble it up. We keep our dogs in a separate area of the kitchen now so they don't get overfed, although escapes do occur.

I have thought a lot about our roles as mum and dad as the boys have grown. Wes is a fantastic father, and he does so much for the babies and is just as capable as I am, but at the same time, there are certain jobs that tend to be left to the woman. I'm the one who organises the weekly shop, who checks what's in the fridge, who prepares Sophia's meals, books medical appointments and keeps on top of the children's vaccinations, as well as the dogs' vet visits and booster shots. I think perhaps there's a certain belief that women are somehow better at admin. I'm not complaining, just stating facts! And while technology makes our lives easier – thank goodness for online shopping – it also complicates things. There's the constant pressure of replying to work emails, answering calls and responding to friends' texts, welcome though they are. I don't know about you, but I always feel guilty if it takes me days to reply to messages.

There was a freedom to being a parent in the era before technology that definitely doesn't exist now. It just adds an extra layer of complexity to an already busy pace of life. One day when Mum was at our house, as she is every day, and I was giving Sophia a drink of water while cleaning the kitchen and prepping bottles for the boys at the same time, Mum piped up, 'Rosie, can you give me a hand with my laptop?'

I said, 'Mum, I haven't got the mental space!'

We laugh about it now, but I realise that we simply have too many demands on our attention. I'm generally able to absorb a lot of pressure, take on plenty of different jobs and multitask well, but even that was too much for me. It's the chaos of being a modern parent.

Wes takes his parenting role of entertainer seriously, and if Sophia is being fussy while I feed her, I'll tell Wes to come over and distract her with funny faces and noises. In fact, one day, he appeared in a blue curly wig to cheer Sophia up because she was in pain from teething. She immediately exploded in laughter and I had to tell him to take it easy or she wouldn't go to bed! And with three children, bedtime is a serious, lengthy business. We don't call the hour before-hand 'The Witching Hour' for nothing. In fact, 5–8 p.m. is absolute chaos, with Sophia's 5.30 p.m. dinner coinciding with the boys' evening bottles. Everyone is tired and grizzly, there's often baby sick on the floor and a nappy explosion to clean up, and Sophia is busy chucking food off her table for the dogs, who then get overexcited and yap incessantly. She's now eating her main meals with a fork and spoon, then snacking on pieces of apple and watermelon, boxes of raisins or slices of toast and butter. She's a great eater, but she's developed a cheeky little habit of hiding food in her high chair, so when I lift her out, there's a shower of food and crumbs.

And if it's bath night, we can definitely prepare for chaos and commotion! They all love having a soak in the tub – especially Sophia, who tries to eat the bubble bath then sprays us with her submarine bath toy. I'll get her out and dry her off before wrapping her up in a little white fluffy dressing-gown, and we take it in turns to bring her up to bed, cosy in her jammies and sleeping bag. It reminds me so much of the noisy fun of my own childhood, having baths with my brothers, splashing around and blowing bubbles, then snuggling up under the duvet while Mum read us a bedtime story.

The twins can be much trickier to settle to sleep, especially now that they're teething. We had just managed to reach the end of our battle with colic and reflux before their gums began to cause them pain, especially at night-time. It can often take up to an hour to soothe them to sleep, with the help of white noise, teething gel and a lot of gentle rocking. To be perfectly honest, it's really draining and the part of the day we both tend to dread, when everyone is tired. They're great babies during the daytime and follow predictable nap patterns but can become overtired and overstimulated by early evening. When we're an hour into them roaring crying, it can be easy to feel frustrated and despondent as a parent. Even though I know the pain they're going through is beyond our control, I can still feel like I'm a bad mum for not being able to make it better and I really have to fight my feelings of guilt and inadequacy. All you want is to do your best for your children, but it's not about being the perfect parent. What matters most is the everyday moments of motherhood, when you're simply being their mum and sharing with them the most precious gift you can give – your time.

When they are all finally tucked up in bed, blissful silence reigns in the house. All is generally calm for a few hours, before the whole cycle begins again and the boys have their 'dream feed' at about 11 p.m. before settling down for the night. It should be time for Netflix or catching up on the news, but I often find myself folding laundry or fitting in a final flurry of emails, all the while reminding myself of the importance of 'self-care'. I think the phrase can be a bit of a marketing buzzword, but I know that it's vital to have time to relax and unwind, even if nowadays that means something small. Before I had children, 'self-care' meant going on holiday, out for a meal or going to a spa – self-indulgent luxuries that seemed entirely normal when Wes and I didn't have children. But now, 'self-care' is far more simple and attainable, yet I appreciate it even more. It's washing my hair with a nice shampoo, having a cup of coffee without it going cold, or doing my nails. It's become about simple tasks where I can just focus on myself for a few minutes. Even eating a meal has become an important little bit of 'me time' at the end of a hectic day, when I've been powered by caffeine and snacks on the go.

The topic of maternal mental and emotional health has developed into an area of interest for me since Sophia was born. Obviously, a father's well-being is just as important, but I can only really comment from my own experiences and perspective. I certainly know that Wes longed to be a dad for many years and he adores his children, but he's found it challenging at times to adapt to life as a parent, particularly in the midst of a global pandemic. Being home from work during the rolling lockdowns of 2020–2021 has given him precious family time, but he's found it difficult on occasion to adapt to his business being closed. He's very driven and ambitious and it can feel disempowering for someone to suddenly be deprived of the stimulation and satisfaction that going to work and supporting your family can bring. He's essentially had to re-evaluate his purpose and everyday role in the home, albeit temporarily until he's permitted to reopen. Like me, he's found solace and sanity through regular home workouts and looked forward to little treats like a Friday-night takeaway or a decent Netflix series. He's been very supportive of my work commitments and I tend to expect a lot from him because he's so capable, but I'm conscious to remind myself frequently that the birth of the boys during a time of huge upheaval has been mentally, emotionally and physically exhausting for him too.

I found pregnancy to be a deeply empowering experi-ence. I loved watching my body change and grow with each passing week – and everything seems to grow even more quickly in a twin pregnancy. I must admit that it made me feel like my body had finally fulfilled its purpose. I found every development fascinating, from my darkening nipples and the emergence of my linea nigra to my wild, vivid dreams and sharpened sense of smell. Seeing how much I was strug-gling from just before the third trimester onwards with basic household tasks, like carrying loads of laundry, cooking, bathing Sophia and bringing the dogs for a walk, Wes took on the majority of physical chores around our home and encouraged me to rest as much as I could. We took Sophia to Dublin Zoo for the first time on 17 September 2020 to celebrate Wes's birthday. I was twenty-six weeks pregnant and we walked for hours, showing her the giraffes, elephants and an array of exotic animals and birds (incidentally, the ducks on the pond were her favourite!). I woke up the next day with swollen, aching feet and lower back pain from the sheer weight in my womb, and it was then we realised that I would have to rest more and avoid walking for any longer than short strolls around the garden. A few of my friends have experienced debilitating pelvic girdle pain in pregnancy, and with an energetic baby to look after, I was keen to avoid that.

What also struck me during my pregnancy and in the weeks and months after the boys' birth is that as a pregnant woman (and especially with twins) you're given a lot of care and attention from medical professionals, family and friends. When your baby (or babies) arrive, the attention is naturally turned to ensuring that they're healthy, happy and well cared for. All of this is completely understandable, and it's human nature to look after the smallest and weakest among us. Yet it's a particularly vulnerable time for new parents, and especially new mums, recovering from the pregnancy and birth and trying to adapt to the enormous mental, emotional and physical upheaval to their lives. As a new mum, you desperately want to do your best for your baby and any encouragement from others means the world to you. To be told that you're doing a wonderful job is all you really want to hear when you're feeling sleep-deprived, hormonal and anxious. The best way to support a new mum, in my experience, is to simply be there for them to offer a hot homemade meal, a cup of tea, the chance to take a nap for an hour, a hand with the laundry or just a sympathetic ear. I've heard some lovely stories of friends and family all putting money towards hiring a night nurse for a night to give new parents a much-needed rest, and there's no better gift, in my opinion. And don't be afraid to ask for help from a family member, friend or medical professional if you're feeling low. It doesn't mean you're weak: it means you're human and normal. I've had to frequently remind myself that I can do anything but not everything as a mum, and that in itself is liberating. As the saying goes, it takes a village to raise a child.

Motherhood is not all baby snuggles, gummy grins and relaxed coffee dates with other mums as popular culture would have us believe. It's joyous for so many wonderful reasons, and I still feel an enormous sense of relief that our battle with infertility is over. Those magical first smiles do bring you incomparable pride and happiness, but it's hard work too, and it's not always rewarding. Newborns are notoriously demanding, and keeping them fed, safe, clean, healthy and happy can feel like relentlessly hard work with little in return. I barely remember the first three or four months with the twins now because we were fuelled by caffeine and adrenaline in a haze of sleep deprivation, baby meltdowns and three-hour feeding cycles. To be perfectly honest, some days and nights were miserable, especially when the boys were tormented with colic and reflux. Yet it feels taboo to say anything negative about your experience of motherhood, especially if you had a difficult road to get there. I felt guilty for complaining about being tired and fed up some days because I had so desperately wanted them – my family was complete. But it's so important to find a way to vent frustration and reduce cortisol levels for your mental and physical health. My poor mum heard a lot of complaints from me in the early months about how the boys wouldn't settle at the same time or kept waking each other up. She always reminded me that everything is just a passing phase with babies and not to take their crying personally. My default reaction to constant, hysterical crying is to blame myself for not being able to soothe them and feel that I'm doing something wrong. I've had to learn that it's their way of communicating and sometimes you can't figure it out – all you can do is hold them and be there with them. But generally, I've found that it's hunger, tiredness, wind, a dirty nappy or sore gums from teething that trigger crying – or a combination!

Quite apart from coping with an unpredictable and demanding little human, it's important to acknowledge the huge changes that happen to your body and your life after you have a baby. Perhaps you're struggling with a changed body shape or stretch marks from pregnancy and breastfeeding, and you don't feel like the old you any more. It can be a frightening loss of identity to not fit into your old clothes or recognise yourself in the mirror, and I can understand the resentment that some new mums feel towards their partners

Some days, while we're sitting at home on our sofa giving the twins yet another bottle feed, Wes and I reminisce about our old life. We love our children beyond words and wouldn't change a thing, but we're comfortable admitting that we miss the freedom, travel and spontaneity of our life before babies. I think it's important to acknowledge that you can be grateful for your family at the same time as wishing you could experience elements of your previous life again, even for a day or two. Whenever I feel myself becoming overwhelmed with the demands of motherhood, I remind myself that the experience of infertility was a million times more exhausting and stressful. As a parent, I believe it's important to figure out what triggers feelings of anxiety and frustration and establish practical ways to cope. I've found it very tough to deal with the incessant crying that comes with colic or teething pain because it's my job to soothe and protect my babies, and I become upset when I can't resolve it. Deep breathing, meditation and mindfulness have been useful tools for remaining calm and collected under challenging circumstances, and I rely almost daily on the healing power of nature. During the first three months with the boys, when I was trying so hard to recover from childbirth, get back to work and cope with having three babies to look after, I would often spend days on end indoors because I simply didn't have the time to step outside for some fresh air. As somebody who has always been happiest in nature, I soon began to feel anxious and lethargic. Going for a walk and spending time outdoors is my most effective coping mechanism – and it's free! I make it a priority to go outside every day now, and I've become much better at postponing or turning down work commitments if I feel they're taking up too much time away from my children. Motherhood has given me a deeper tenacity, strength and resolve than ever before because my children need my attention and energy now. Anything that threatens to waste it is removed from my life. It's taught me a lot about priorities, to leave my phone aside, deal with other distractions such as emails or phone calls at a later time, and give them my full attention. Every day, something new and different happens with one of them – Sophia taking her first steps, Hugo giggling at me as I tickle him, Oscar trying to pull himself up to a seated position on the playmat – and when it does I remind myself that I won't see this again: they're constantly growing and changing. I don't want to miss out on special moments with them and all of this goes back to the importance of looking after yourself as a parent to be physically and psychologically strong enough to care for others.

As for so many people, lockdown has given me time to reflect. When there are no distractions, you really do tend to focus on what matters most in life. And I believe that what matters most is family and our health. My absolute priority is the children, to make sure that they are happy, fed, comfortable and cuddled – everything else can wait. Wes and I have so many plans to give them the most magical childhood.

He can't wait for the day when we bring them to Disneyland and we have lots of special dreams for us as a family, but we know that it's the small things they'll really remember. I can clearly remember occasions when I was a child like Mum's birthday, when we all celebrated by snuggling up to her in bed, eating chocolate biscuits. She probably just wanted the morning off mum duty, but we thought it was great fun being allowed to eat snacks under the duvet! When I reflect on my childhood, I have so many small but significant recollections: hours spent running around the garden, building a fort from sofa cushions in the living room on rainy days, eating hot, salty chipper chips drenched in vinegar on a Friday night and cheese on toast on Sunday evenings. It was probably Mum's way of not having to plan and cook a meal for once, but we thought it was just the best thing ever. I want our kids to do the same and to build their own happy memories.

Sometimes I wonder what our lives would have been like if our family dreams hadn't come true. I think back to what Wes said about how we'd still have a meaningful life, and of course we would. Plenty of people have to come to terms with exactly that: their life hasn't turned out the way they had planned and they make the very best of it. Wes and I would have done that too, although it would have been a painful process, and every day I appreciate how lucky we are that we have our family.

Almost daily, Wes will say, 'I can't believe we have three children.' I know exactly what he means. We were just getting used to the idea of having Sophia in our lives when a miracle happened and I became pregnant with twins. I think it'll take a while longer for us to get our heads around it and adapt to our new status. But there was a moment when we were in the kitchen and Wes was grabbing a cup of coffee for both of us while I was giving Sophia her breakfast. The boys were in their twin chair gurgling and all five of us, including the dogs, were pottering about, and I said, 'Could you ever have imagined it? A family of five.' Every time I say the words, I'm surprised by them.

Here we are and look at where we've come from. We are no longer that couple at weddings and christenings unable to have a family of our own. I don't feel that ache of sadness any more as I congratulate a friend on a pregnancy or welcome her new baby into the world with a little gift. Now I can join in conversations on teething and feeding schedules and share parenting stories with other mums. But I'll never forget what we went through to have our family.

As I said right at the beginning of this book, one of the reasons I wrote it is for my children to read in years to come and for them to understand how much we wanted them and how very much we love them. Perhaps they'll show it to their own children too.

But this book is also for everyone who has experienced the heartbreak and lost innocence of infertility, miscarriage and stillbirth. And it's to offer strength and hope to those of you who will face it in the future. When Wes and I were battling through the multiple miscarriages, I had plenty of support, but I didn't have anyone I could turn to who had experienced anything similar. I used to trawl through internet chat pages and pregnancy websites to gather information and read about other people's success stories. I needed to know that fertility miracles could happen. I would have loved to find a book like this to answer some of my many questions and for reassurance that things can and do work out. I hope that it's been of some value and comfort to you and, most of all, that your own wishes and dreams come true.

Lots of love,
Rosanna